YOUR INJURY

A COMMON SENSE GUIDE TO SPORTS INJURIES

Merrill A. Ritter, M.D. & Marjorie J. Albohm, A.T., C.

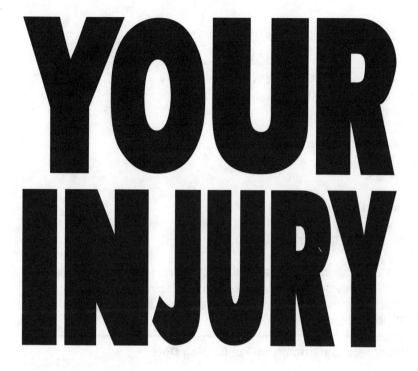

MASTERS PRESS

A Division of Howard W. Sams & Co.

Trade edition published by Masters Press, 1994
(A Division of Howard W. Sams & Co.)
2647 Waterfront Pkwy. E. Drive, Suite 300
Indianapolis, IN 46214

© 1987, Cooper Publishing Group
P.O. Box 562
Carmel, IN 46032

Library of Congress Cataloging-in-Publication Data

Ritter, Merrill A.

    Your injury: a common sense guide to sports injuries/ Merrill A. Ritter, Marjorie J. Albohm.

      p. cm.

    Previous ed. published: Indianapolis : Benchmark Press, 1987.

    ISBN 1-57028-011-8

    1. Sports Injuries--Handbooks, manuals, etc. 2. Sports injuries -- Prevention--Handbooks, manuals, etc. I. Albohm, Marjorie J. II. Title.

RD97.R57 1994	94-16249
617.1'027--dc20	CIP

Credits:

Art: Craig Gosling

Cover Design: Suzanne Lincoln

How To Use This Book

This book was written for the avid athlete, the weekend jogger, and the first-aid specialist—in short, anyone who could be confronted with injuries caused by physical activity. It is designed for quick reference, yet it provides ample information to support prompt, sensible decisions.

Readers should review Chapters 1 through 4, which provide background information and general advice about injury identification and management. Any person who supervises or participates in athletic activities should be familiar with this material.

The remaining 14 chapters describe common injuries in specific parts of the body. The injury sections include information on Symptoms; Do's, (actions to take to solve the problem); Don'ts (actions to avoid); and Modifications (changes to make to promote healing and maintain conditioning in the rest of the body).

Each chapter concludes with a series of exercise descriptions. The modifications direct readers to perform certain exercises which are identified by numbers and designed to help strengthen specific areas.

Following the guidelines in this book will enable you to treat most sports injuries properly, consult a physician when necessary, and—most importantly—resume activities safely.

The following terms appear often in the text and are defined here for your convenience.

Bursa: A pad-like sac, found around joints, which contain fluid. Bursae reduce friction caused by movements of tendons and ligaments.

Disc: A rigid cartilage substance containing a jelly-like center that sits between each vertebra in the back. Its purpose is to absorb shock.

Dislocation: Movement of a bone completely out of its normal position in a joint.

Extension: Movement of a body part away from the rest of the body part into a straightened position.

Flexion: Movement of a body part toward the rest of the body into a bent position.

Hyperextension: Extreme or abnormal straightening of a body part beyond normal extension.

Ligament: A band of strong tissue which holds one end of a bone to another so the joint will not come apart.

Spasm: An involuntary sudden movement or muscular contraction.

Subluxation: Movement of a bone partially out of its normal position in a joint and back into its proper location.

Tendon: That portion of a muscle that narrows into a thick band before it attaches to the bone.

Vertebra: A bony segment of the spinal column.

Your Injury Guide

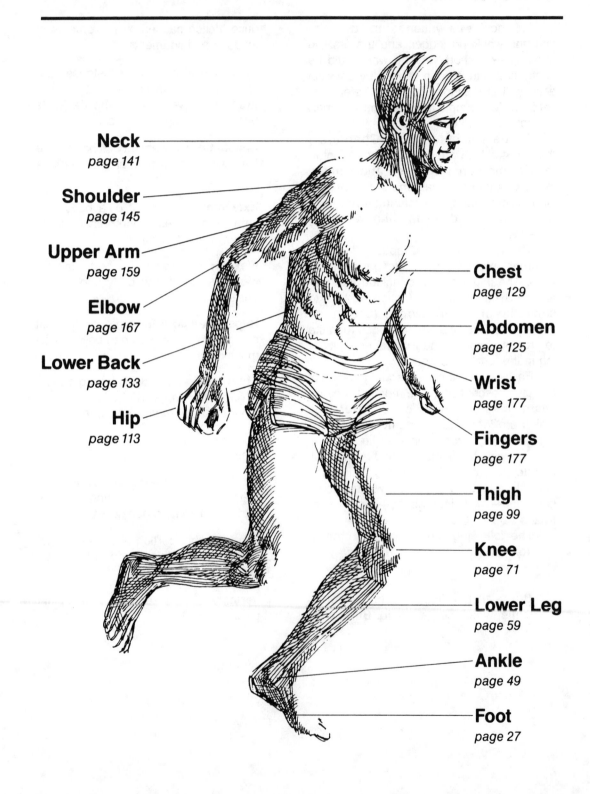

Neck
page 141

Shoulder
page 145

Upper Arm
page 159

Elbow
page 167

Lower Back
page 133

Hip
page 113

Chest
page 129

Abdomen
page 125

Wrist
page 177

Fingers
page 177

Thigh
page 99

Knee
page 71

Lower Leg
page 59

Ankle
page 49

Foot
page 27

TABLE OF CONTENTS

CHAPTER 16: THE UPPER ARM 159

CHAPTER 17: THE ELBOW 167

CHAPTER 18: THE WRIST AND FINGERS 177

DEDICATIONS

To my wife, Nanette, my daughter, Wendy, and my son, Jake, who have withstood the absence of their husband and father over many years of hard work while in the field of medicine. Medicine is a specialty which requires a great dedication not only of yourself, but of your family. Their understanding and love allowed me to take care of others as well as them. To them I dedicate this book.

Merrill A. Ritter, M.D.

For my friend Priscilla, and all the other everyday athletes who love to be active and who deserve to be injury free. To my co-author Merrill Ritter, who inspires me to believe that each goal and dream is attainable and that reaching for them is exciting.

Marjorie J. Albohm, A.T.,C.

ACKNOWLEDGEMENTS

The authors gratefully acknowledge the following people who made this publication possible: Craig Gosling, Director of Medical Illustrations, Indiana University School of Medicine, and his staff; Artists Lydia Kibiuk and John Nixon; Photographers John Murphy and David Jaynes; Designer Gary Schmitt; Models Abby Marmion and Bill Marrocco; Manuscript preparation, Beth Divine.

FOREWORD

Experts have vividly described the benefits of regular exercise. As Americans have heeded the advice and headed for running tracks, swimming pools, and basement nautilus machines, they have occasionally fallen prey to sports injuries—the sprained ankles, dislocated thumbs, and tennis elbows that come from overuse, mistakes, and plain bad luck.

There is good news. Two respected Indiana authorities, Merrill A. Ritter, M.D., and Marjorie J. Albohm, A.T.,C., wrote this book to help sidelined athletes of all ages and abilities identify their problems, repair the damage, stay in shape while healing, and resume activities.

These first-rate scholars and practitioners have compiled a lucid, well-organized text that should be on the bookshelves of everyday athletes, school nurses, camp directors, parents, and first-aid technicians. With the help of hundreds of clear illustrations and photographs, the authors provide background information on injury management and then describe specific injuries in detail, literally from head to toe. The tone is sensible and encouraging.

As an avid runner, I know that no athlete wants to be out of commission for long. One of the unique aspects of this book is its attention to alternative conditioning methods for use during rehabilitation periods. Physicians and athletic trainers will attest to the merit of the information and advice in this timely book.

I am proud to endorse the work of two fellow Hoosiers, both of whom were educated in Indiana—a state known for its passion for basketball and devotion to amateur athletics. As colleagues at the Indiana University School of Medicine and the International Institute for Sports Science and Medicine, Dr. Ritter and Ms. Albohm contribute greatly to the growing body of knowledge in the field of sports medicine. As advisors to the 1987 Pan American Games in Indianapolis, they will assist athletes from around the world. With this book, they have summarized valuable information for the welfare of citizens dedicated to physical fitness and healthier lives.

Richard G. Lugar
U.S. Senator from Indiana

What is an Injury?

When you are injured you are immediately concerned about the nature of the injury—its complexity, severity, and duration. Some basic information will enable you to better understand the injury. You will be able to recognize key symptoms that indi-cate diagnosis and severity, initiate suitable first aid treatment, modify activity in the appropriate way, and take a common sense approach to the problem.

Chapter 1

What is a Sprain?

A sprain is an injury to a ligament **(Figure 1-1)** which causes pain and disability depending on the degree of the injury. Ligaments tear when stressed excessively **(Figure 1-2)**. When a ligament is torn or stretched, the particular joint it supports becomes loose. The amount of joint instability is sometimes difficult to assess and is best evaluated by a physician.

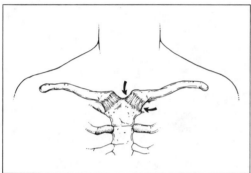

Figure 1-1. Ligament in shoulder attaching collarbone to sternum.

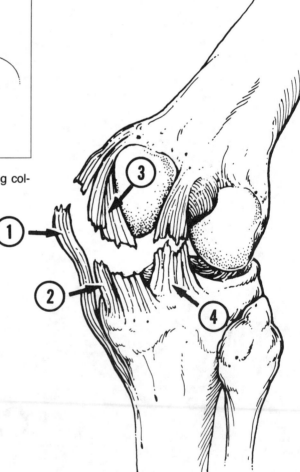

Figure 1-2. Torn ligaments on the inside (1,2,3) and in the middle (4) of the knee (posterior view).

Sprains are classified in degrees, according to the amount of tearing that has occurred in the ligament(s). A mild sprain is a 1st degree sprain with minimal stretching of the ligament fibers and no instability of the joint **(Figure 1-3)**. A moderate sprain is a 2nd degree sprain with more but not complete tearing. There is some instability of the joint, but the ligament is still intact **(Figure 1-4)**. A severe sprain is a 3rd degree sprain with the ligament totally torn in two or more pieces. The joint is unstable **(Figure 1-5)**.

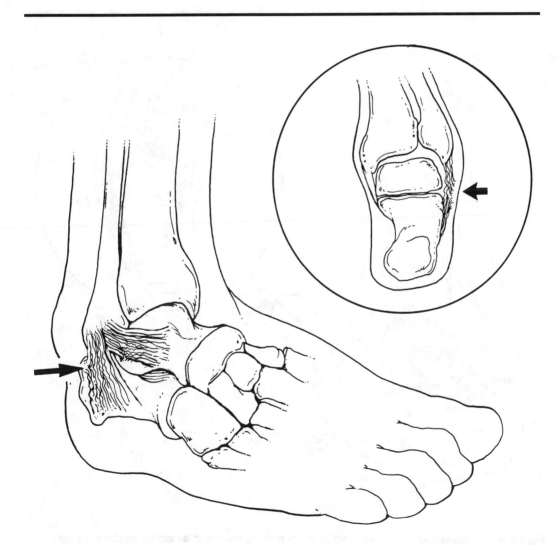

Figure 1-3. Mild, 1st degree sprain of the outside ligaments in an ankle. Inset shows view from behind ankle.

First and 2nd degree sprains are treated by conservative measures such as rest, ice, compression, elevation, and support. Specific reconditioning exercises are appropriate so that the muscles surrounding the injured joint do not weaken. General exercises may be continued and are frequently recommended for these injuries if the stress of the exercise does not separate the previously torn ligament. Use common sense—avoid activities that are painful to the injured area. *Remember, healing takes 6 to 12 weeks.*

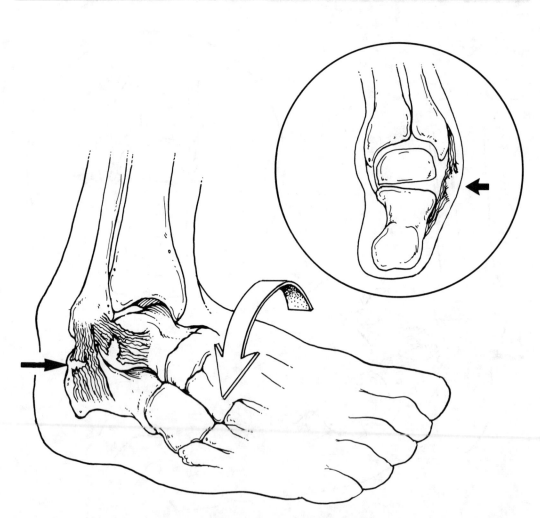

Figure 1-4. Moderate, 2nd degree sprain of the outside ligaments in an ankle. Inset shows view from behind ankle.

Third degree sprains frequently require surgical repair. Examination by a physician will determine the degree of ligament injury. Ligaments do not show on x-rays, which are often necessary to rule out any bone injury.

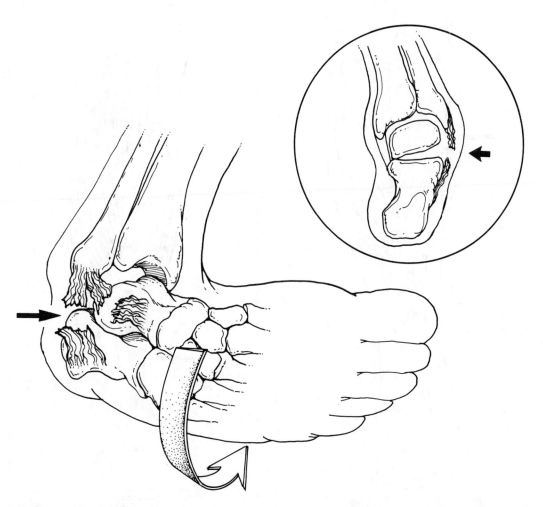

Figure 1-5. Severe, 3rd degree sprain of the outside ligaments in an ankle. Inset shows view from behind ankle.

What is a Strain?

A strain is tearing of muscle tissue either in the main part of the muscle or in the tendon unit **(Figure 1-6)**. This injury produces pain and disability, depending upon the extent of the tear.

Strains, like sprains, are classified by degrees. A mild, 1st degree strain involves minimal muscle tearing **(Figure 1-7)**. A moderate, 2nd degree strain involves more muscle tearing **(Figure 1-8)**. A severe, 3rd degree strain involves a total tear and separation of the muscle allowing no active muscle function to move the joint where the tendon attaches **(Figure 1-9)**. This is sometimes referred to as a rupture.

The 1st and 2nd degree strains are treated conservatively with rest, ice, compression, elevation, and support. Certain reconditioning exercises may also be appropriate. A 3rd degree strain requires

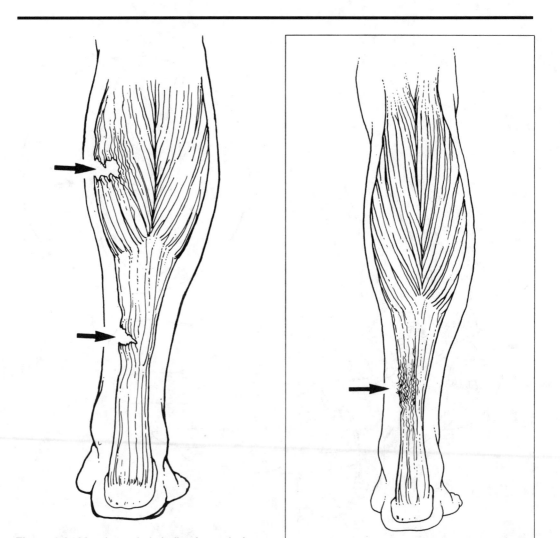

Figure 1-6. Muscle strain in belly of muscle (upper) and in muscle tendon unit (lower).

Figure 1-7. Mild, 1st degree muscle strain in muscle tendon unit.

specific medical attention. Muscle tissue and tendons, like ligaments, do *not* show up on x-rays. A physician can determine the severity of the muscle injury.

General exercises may be continued if the injured area is allowed to rest and heal. Use common sense—exercising an injured muscle will delay healing. Therefore, do only those exercises that do not affect the injured area.

Muscle injuries take a long time to heal. It is not unusual to have symptoms linger 6 months or more depending on severity of the injury.

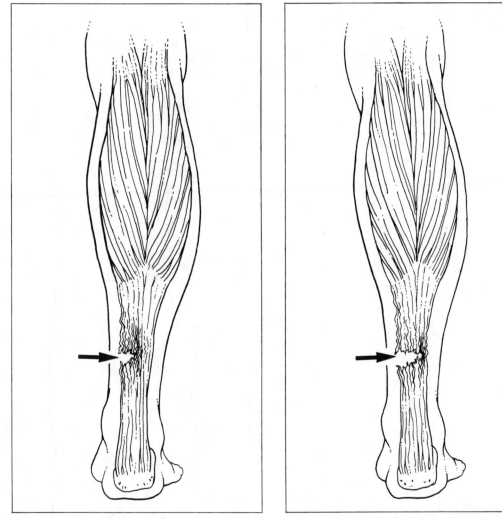

Figure 1-8. Moderate, 2nd degree muscle strain in muscle tendon unit.

Figure 1-9. Severe, 3rd degree muscle strain in muscle tendon unit.

What is a Contusion?

A contusion is another word for a bruise. It is a local area of bleeding beneath the skin caused by the rupture of blood vessels related to a direct blow or tearing of tissue **(Figure 1-10)**. The size of the bruise only reflects the amount of bleeding, not necessarily the severity of the injury.

If the bruise is very deep within a muscle, the discoloration may not surface and therefore may not be visible. Bruises vary in size, and in most cases, severity depends upon the nature of the contact or blow.

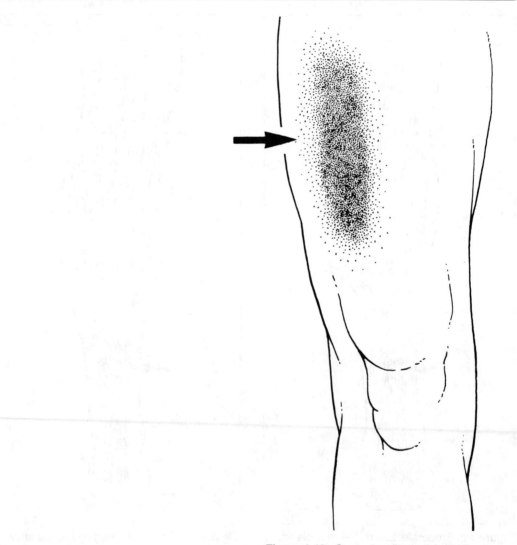

Figure 1-10. Contusion (bruise) in thigh.

What is a Fracture?

A fracture is a break of a bone into 2 or more pieces as a result of an injury. There are several types of fractures: stress, avulsion, closed, and open.

A stress fracture is an area in a bone that is about to break but has not. It is not necessarily due to an injury, but it may be caused by one **(Figure 1-11)**. An avulsion fracture is a fragment of bone pulled off its original location by a supporting ligament or tendon **(Figure 1-12)**. A closed fracture, also known as a simple fracture, is a broken

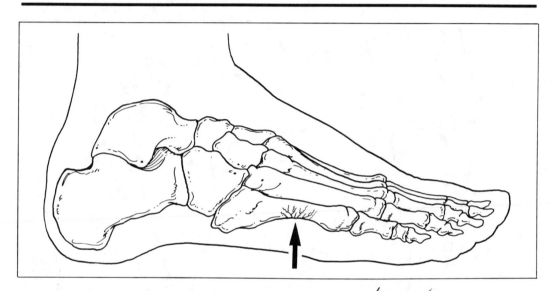

Figure 1-11. Stress fracture in 5th metatarsal bone in foot.

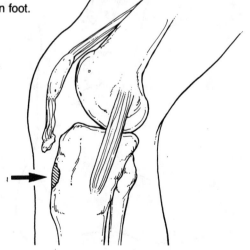

Figure 1-12. Avulsion fracture in knee.

bone in which the skin has not been punctured **(Figure 1-13)**. An open fracture, also known as a compound fracture, occurs when the broken bones have poked through the skin **(Figure 1-14)**.

If you are told you have a fracture, you will want to know the type, whether it is complete or incomplete, and whether or not it will need to be reduced (placed in correct alignment) before casting. A complete fracture is when a bone is broken all the way through. An incomplete fracture is when a bone is broken partially through. Regardless of type or size, all breaks in bones are fractures. Avulsion, closed, and open fractures are visible on x-rays. Stress fractures, however, may not show up on an x-ray for 3 to 6 weeks.

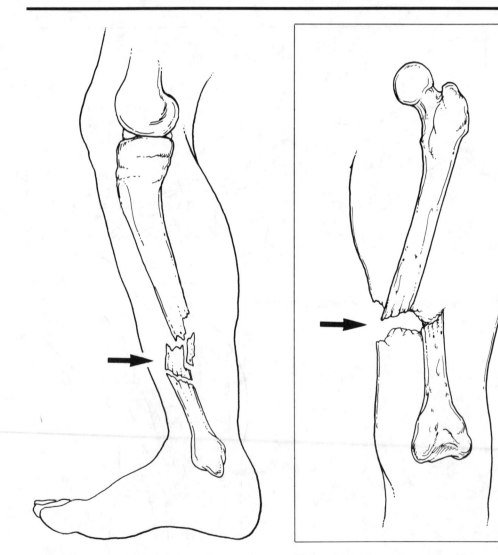

Figure 1-13. Closed fracture in lower leg.

Figure 1-14. Open fracture in thigh.

What is a Dislocation?

A dislocation is the temporary removal of a bone from its normal position in a joint **(Figure 1-15)**. This can be caused by a direct force or an extreme movement beyond a joint's normal range of motion. When a bone is dislocated, ligaments and muscle tendons are torn, allowing the bone and the joint to come apart.

Dislocations can occur in any joint in the body, but they are more common at the shoulder, elbow, fingers, and kneecap. All dislocations are extremely painful until the bones are back in their normal positions. This repositioning or reducing *should only be done by a physician*.

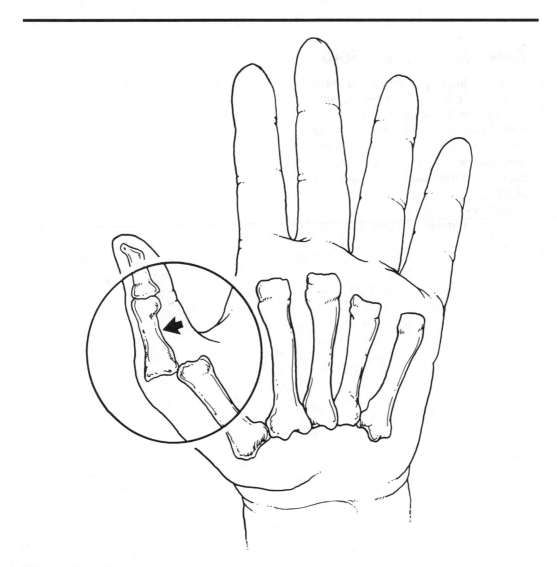

Figure 1-15. Dislocated thumb.

Acute versus Chronic

An acute injury is an injury that has just happened or is only a few days old. A chronic problem is one which has lasted several weeks. Often, a chronic problem does not get any better or any worse, but continues to exist.

Overuse can cause chronic problems to worsen and become acute. A stress fracture is a good example. The previously injured area is pushed beyond its limits, and an acute fracture occurs. This often happens when one overtrains or trains too hard while compensating for another injury.

In an acute injury you will remember a specific incident that caused the difficulty.

Seeking Further Help

Sometimes it is difficult to know what specific injury you have and what you should do about it. This book should enable you to better evaluate or identify most injuries and take appropriate action. If you are ever in doubt about the severity or proper care of an injury, or if particular symptoms persist for more than 3 to 5 days, see a physician or medical specialist in your area.

Proper, Immediate First Aid

When you have an injury, there is going to be sudden (acute) swelling. This is due to bleeding in and around the injured area, inflammation (the body's response to injury) or both. If swelling is controlled and minimized, the injured area is less painful, and motion and rehabilitation can begin sooner. Swelling is best controlled by rest, ice, compression, and elevation (R.I.C.E.).

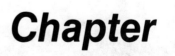

Chapter **2**

Rest

Resting an injured area is one of the best treatments. Healing progresses more rapidly when stress is reduced. It is only necessary to rest the injured area, however, not the entire body. Continue a general exercise program as long as it is not painful to the injured area. Forms of rest for an injury may include casting, splinting, using crutches or a cane, or any combination of these methods.

Compression

Compression is used to put pressure on an injured area to decrease swelling. It is best applied in the form of a wet elastic bandage. (Using a wet bandage will quickly transmit the cold from an ice pack to the injured area.) The wrap should be applied in a circular pattern starting at a point near the toes or fingers and wrapping toward the body, squeezing gently **(Figure 2-1)**. If a knee is injured and you compress only the knee, then the area from the knee to the foot will swell because the tight bandage prevents fluid from returning to the body.

Ice packs should be applied after the compression wrap is completed.

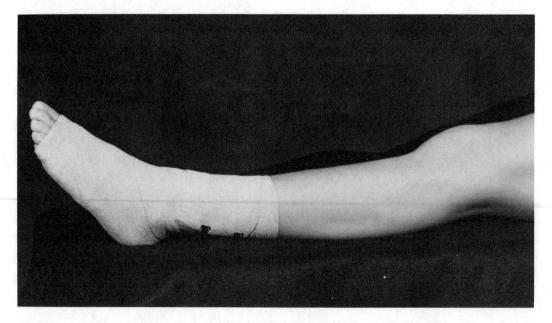

Figure 2-1. Compression wrap starting at the toes and wrapping toward the shin.

Ice

The purpose of using ice is to constrict the blood vessels in an injured area to slow down bleeding. Ice also lessens the tremendous inflammatory reaction of the body to the injury, helps to deaden some of the pain, and allows movement and reconditioning of the injured area to proceed a little faster.

Ice can be applied in a plastic bag, moist towels, commercial cold packs, or any other form available **(Figure 2-2)**.

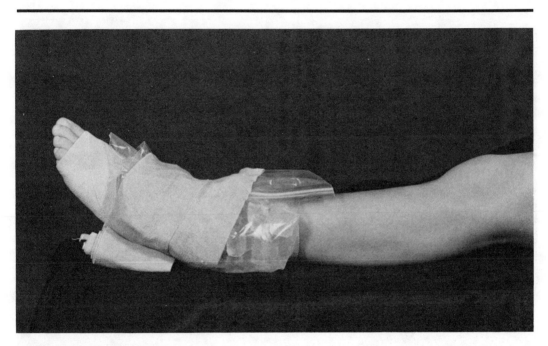

Figure 2-2. Ice packs on ankle.

Elevation

Elevation is also used to inhibit swelling. By elevating an injured body part you are combating the effect of gravity which tends to pull blood and fluids down to the injured area, where they pool.

Elevation is used after the injured area has been compressed with a wet elastic bandage and ice packs have been applied **(Figure 2-3)**.

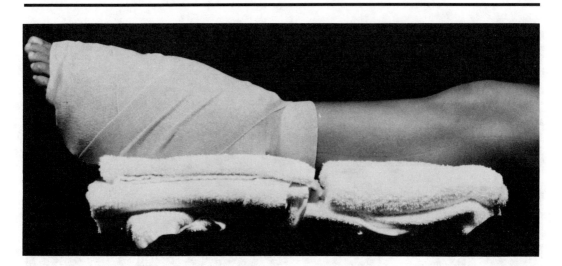

Figure 2-3. Elevation—above hip level.

Treatment Time

The treatment of ice, compression, and elevation should be used for 20 to 30 minutes at a time as often as possible during the first 48 to 72 hours after an injury or whenever swelling is present. *DO NOT USE HEAT AT ANY TIME.* Heat increases swelling. There is no place for heat in the treatment of acute injuries and possibly even in chronic injuries. Always use ice unless a medical expert gives you different instructions.

Support

When you are not treating your injury with rest, ice, compression, and elevation, it should be protected by some means of support such as a brace, splint, dry elastic bandage, adhesive tape, or similar device **(Figure 2-4)**.

Remember, for a new injury (acute) or the recurrence of swelling, use *rest, ice, compression* and *elevation*—R.I.C.E.—and keep the injured area supported and protected at all times.

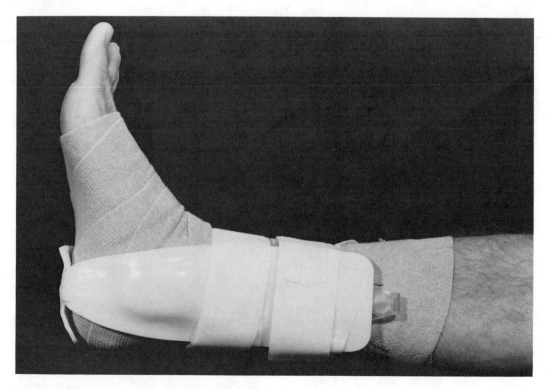

Figure 2-4. Wrap and brace support of an ankle.

Principles of Rehabilitation

Rehabilitation is one of the most important phases of handling an injury, yet it is frequently overlooked. Rehabilitation is the restoration of an injured or weakened area to a normal healthy state through the use of specific exercises, designed to strengthen the muscles that surround the injured area.

Without rehabilitation, an injured body area will remain weak, and the likelihood of injury recurrence is great. It is essential to rehabilitate all injuries, from the most minor to the most severe.

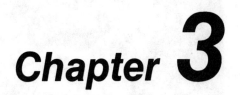

Chapter **3**

The principles that apply to conditioning also apply to rehabilitation. Exercises specific to a given area must be performed, and the exercises must become progressively harder for improvement to occur and for the muscles to get stronger.

The difference between conditioning and rehabilitation is that in rehabilitation the focus is on an injured area. The resistance is lower, and the number of repetitions is fewer. The goal is to restore the injured area to its original condition without hampering the healing process.

While rehabilitating an injured area, it is important to prevent deconditioning of the total body. Maintaining overall strength, flexibility, endurance, and coordination is essential. Many total body exercises such as swimming, biking, and weight training can be continued during rehabilitation to keep the total body in condition. Any exercise can be performed as long as it does not cause stress, pain, or discomfort to the injured area.

Immediately following injury, the treatment of rest, ice, compression, and elevation (R.I.C.E.) should be applied (see Chapter 2). When the swelling has been controlled and there is not severe pain, rehabilitation may be started. It may begin with isometric-type exercises, which involve strengthening muscles without movement of the body part. These can be performed even if the area is immobilized in a cast. When more movement is possible, exercises are added to take the body part through as much of its normal range of motion as is comfortable **(Figure 3-1 and 2)**.

Figure 3-1 and 2. Range of motion exercise for the foot and ankle (point, then flex).

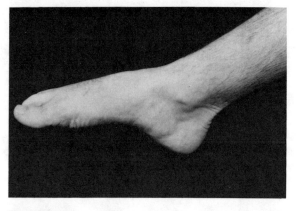

Figure 3-1.

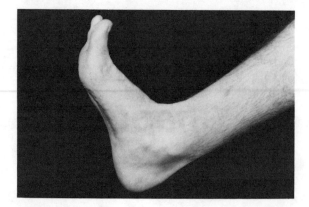

Figure 3-2.

When normal movement is restored, resistance can be added **(Figure 3-3)**. This makes the muscles in the area work harder and become stronger. As the muscles adjust to a particular level, additional resistance must be applied for continued strengthening to occur.

Initial rehabilitation exercises are usually done in short bouts (20 to 30 repetitions), repeated 2 to 3 times daily. As resistance is added, the intensity increases, and exercises are performed fewer times, (only once or twice a day).

Doing too much rehabilitative exercise or working with too much resistance will cause pain and possibly additional swelling in the injured area. This could decrease the normal movement in the joint and decrease the strengthening effect that you are trying to produce. Do not, at any time, perform rehabilitation exercises if they cause pain.

The injury is fully rehabilitated when complete normal motion is present, swelling is absent, and the previously injured area feels and looks as strong as the corresponding non-injured part. All physical activity can be performed without pain or limitations in movement.

The exercises found at the end of each chapter may be used as conditioning exercises, to prevent injury, or as rehabilitation exercises to regain strength following injury.

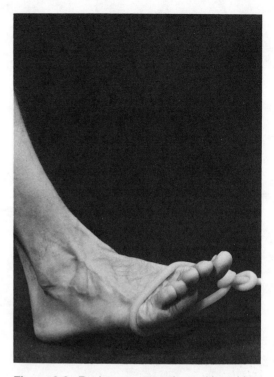

Figure 3-3. Resistance exercise with rubber tubing for the foot and ankle.

Environmental Concerns

Exercising in very hot, humid weather or in very cold, windy weather presents some potential problems and dangers. You should always be aware of the environmental conditions surrounding physical activity.

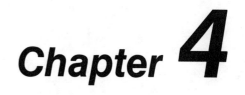

Chapter **4**

Heat-Related Problems

The body is cooled primarily through the evaporation of sweat. Warm temperatures increase sweating, but the effectiveness of sweat evaporation depends heavily on the relative humidity present. High humidity levels reduce the rate of evaporation without reducing the rate of sweating. Therefore, when high temperatures and high humidity are present, sweat is not evaporated easily, the body is not cooled, and heat problems are likely to occur. This is similar to what can happen to a person exercising in a rubber suit that does not let sweat evaporate.

Types of Heat Problems

Heat problems may exist in the form of heat cramps, heat exhaustion, or heat stroke.

Heat cramps are muscle cramps (spasms, twitching) that occur in several locations in the body, usually during or immediately after heavy exertion in hot, humid weather. When they occur, you should stop activity, move to a cool, shaded area, and drink water to replace fluids lost through sweating. In most cases activity can be resumed the following day.

Heat exhaustion may have varied symptoms. Again, it usually takes place during or immediately after strenuous work in hot, humid weather. A person may feel nauseated, disoriented, and/or weak. The skin is usually cool and clammy. Muscles may feel weak and tired, and they do not function in a coordinated manner. You know there is something wrong, but you may not be sure what it is. With any of these symptoms, move to a cool, shaded area; drink water to replace fluids lost through sweat; and rest. Avoid any physical activity for a day or two until all of the symptoms have disappeared.

Heat stroke is a sudden failure of the thermoregulatory system. It is a life-threatening problem with a very rapid onset. It occurs during extreme activity in hot, humid weather. The victim does not sweat, and the skin is hot, flushed, and dry. The individual usually goes into shock and is unconscious. Call emergency assistance immediately, and get the person to a hospital. Lower the body temperature any way possible. Spray the person with a garden hose, or submerge the person in cold water.

Heat stroke is rare. It is an extremely serious and potentially fatal problem.

Prevention of Heat Problems

- Recognize the temperature and humidity conditions, and take appropriate precautions.
- Replace fluids lost through sweat by drinking water freely.
- Become accustomed to exercising in heat and humidity in steps; begin your exercise program gradually.
- Wear cool clothing—short-sleeved or sleeveless shirts, mesh tops, and shorts.
- Do not exercise during the hottest part of the day.
- Make sure you are taking in enough salt, potassium, and calcium in your diet. These are essential minerals commonly lost through sweat. Manufactured supplements to help prevent heat problems often do more harm than good. Ingesting salt tablets to replace salt lost through sweat is one example. Many times the salt tablets are difficult to digest and therefore the salt never leaves the stomach. In this state they are of no value to the body. Also, too much salt obtained through a large intake of salt tablets may further upset the chemical and electrolyte balance of the body.
- Various sport drinks are manufactured and marketed to aid in fluid replacement and the prevention of heat problems. Often the drinks contain high concentrations of sugar which tend to upset the stomach during and after activity. Also, some persons do not like the taste of the drinks and therefore may not consume enough if sports drinks are the only beverages available. The safest and most accepted fluid replacement is plain water.

Cold-Related Problems

Exercising in cold weather may also present some specific dangers. Low temperatures alone can be a problem, but when wind is present, the chill factor may be critical. A small drop in body temperature can affect neuromuscular responses and may cause muscle fatigue.

Types of Cold Problems

Cold weather problems may include frostnip, superficial frostbite, and deep frostbite.

Frostnip affects the tips of such extremities as the ears, nose, fingers, and toes. This commonly occurs when high winds are present. The skin is firm and cold. It may peel or blister in a day or so. Firm pressure of your hand on the affected area(s) may help.

Superficial frostbite makes the affected area pale, waxy, cold, and hard. It involves only the superficial layers of skin. When the area is rewarming it will first feel numb, then it will sting and burn. Blistering may occur later, and the area may be painful for several weeks.

Deep frostbite is very serious and requires immediate hospitalization. Deep tissues are frozen. The injured area is hard, cold, numb, pale, or white. Medically supervised rapid rewarming is required. During rewarming the skin may become blotchy-red, swollen, and extremely painful.

Prevention of Cold Problems

- Do sufficient warm-up activities prior to exercise, and avoid periods of inactivity while outside.
- Cover the face, nose, ears, and fingers.
- Wear warm headgear. Much heat is lost through an exposed head.
- Wear non-constricting, multi-layer clothing that "breathes" to prevent sweat from accumulating on skin, causing a chilling effect.
- *Do not* put affected areas in cold water or snow. This only makes problems worse.

The Foot

Your foot is a complex unit. It is made of multiple bones, joints, ligaments, and muscles **(Figure 5-1)**. It is designed for flexibility and strength to allow you to perform a variety of weight-bearing activities and coordinated movements. Your feet bear your full body weight, and they balance and transport your body through all types of movement patterns at varying speeds.

There are many structural differences in the feet of individuals, including flat feet, high arches, bunions, claw toes, and calluses. Due to the functions of feet and those differences, many activity-related injuries and conditions occur in the feet. These problems require proper management and *good common sense*.

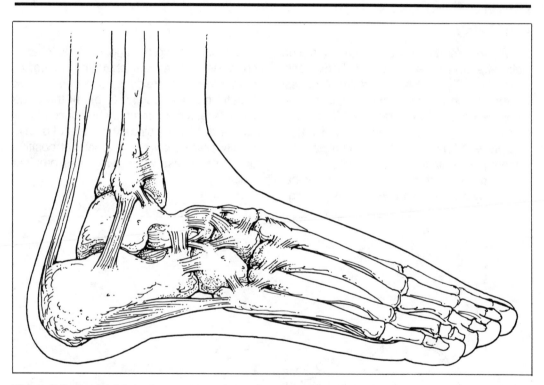

Figure 5-1. Bones, joints, ligaments, and muscles of the foot.

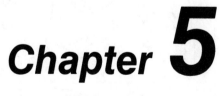

Chapter **5**

If pain in the foot continues and various symptoms get worse, your prospects for putting weight on the foot and staying active are diminished. By properly attending to these problems, you will be able to continue your normal activities.

Pain on/near Bony Area in Foot
(Stress Fracture, March Fracture)

A stress fracture usually occurs in major weight-bearing locations of the body such as the foot **(Figure 5-2)** or the leg. A stress fracture which occurs in the foot is sometimes called a "March fracture." The term gets its name from the common condition in soldiers who begin marching long distances without prior training.

A stress fracture in the foot may be caused by beginning a new activity too vig-orously, increasing training intensity, changing types of surfaces, changing shoes, or returning from a previous injury too quickly. Repetitive stress begins to break the bone down. Stress fractures may be difficult to diagnose accurately since the onset of pain is usually gradual and x-rays are not positive for 3 to 6 weeks after symptoms are first noticed.

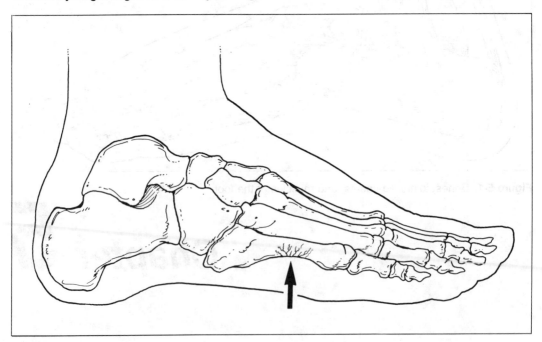

Figure 5-2. Stress fracture in the 5th metatarsal bone of the foot.

Stress fractures in the foot usually occur in the ball of the foot around the 2nd or 3rd toes **(Figure 5-3)** or on the outside of the foot at the base of the little toe (5th metatarsal) **(Figure 5-4)**. A stress fracture in the foot may also be found in the area of the heel bone (os calcis) **(Figure 5-5)**.

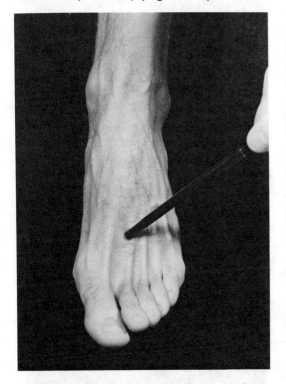

Figure 5-3. Common location of a stress fracture in the ball of the foot.

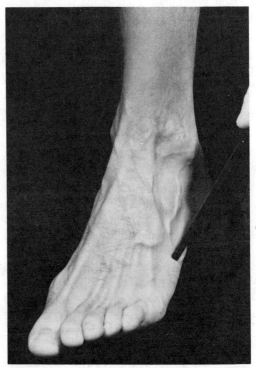

Figure 5-4. Common location of a stress fracture in the 5th metatarsal bone of the foot.

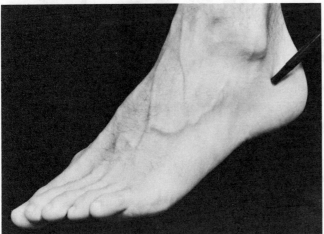

Figure 5-5. Common location of a stress fracture in the heel bone.

Symptoms

Stress fractures are characterized by a gradual onset of pain associated with increased weight-bearing activities, such as running or jumping. This pain is progressive. It will slowly become more intense as the activity is continued. There is usually a specific area of pain (point tenderness) directly over the affected bone. This pain may persist in varying degrees for a period of 4 to 12 weeks. The symptoms gradually subside over time as the bone heals by adapting to the added stress—providing that you change the stressful activity or decrease its intensity.

Do's

- Continue weight-bearing activities (running, jumping) as tolerated only to the point of pain. Decrease or stop these activities if the pain gets worse or does not subside.
- Use ice, compression, and elevation for 20 to 30 minutes following activity or excessive weight bearing.
- All exercises listed at the end of the chapter should be done without an increase in pain.
- Pad or donut the area to reduce the direct pressure on the affected bone **(Figure 5-6)**. This is not to be used if pain persists. Stop the activity instead.
- If pain persists, have the problem evaluated by a physician performing an x-ray and possibly a bone scan, if the x-ray is negative. A bone scan will tell almost immediately if a stress fracture is present.

Don'ts

- Do not ignore this problem. It will worsen progressively. Continued activity may produce a complete fracture.
- Do not continue weight-bearing activities if the degree of pain causes limping or impaired movement.

Modifications

- Pad or donut the affected area to relieve specific pressure.
- Perform non-weight-bearing activities such as bicycling or swimming.
- Crutches may be used if pain is intense.
- Continue weight training for the upper and lower extremities.
- Physicians may prescribe a slipper type cast especially for the fracture on the side of the foot.

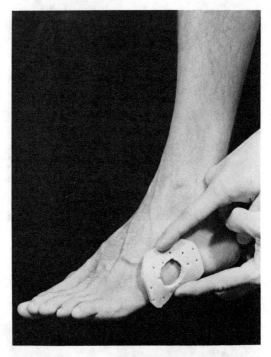

Figure 5-6. Donut pad used to take pressure off affected bone.

Pain on Heel
(Heel Bruise, Stone Bruise)

A heel bruise is usually related to a direct impact on the bottom of the heel from such activities as jumping or landing inadvertently on the heel instead of the toes. The heel's heavy pad of tissue for protection is not always enough cushion. The bone itself, the cushion, or both may become bruised.

Symptoms

Symptoms of this problem are specific pain in the heel region and extreme pain in the heel when bearing weight. There is a feeling that a stone or foreign body may be in the shoe putting pressure on the heel when you step down. One spot on the bottom of the heel is very tender **(Figure 5-7)**.

Do's

- Use rest, ice, compression, and elevation for 20 to 30 minutes after activity or excessive weight bearing.
- Use an ice cup as shown in **(Figure 5-8)**. Apply in small circular motions until ice is gone.
- Pad or donut the area to relieve the specific pressure on the point of irritation **(Figure 5-9)**.
- Continue weight-bearing activities as tolerated to the point of pain.

Don'ts

- Do not use heat, as it will increase soreness by causing more swelling.
- Avoid excessive weight bearing or jumping directly on the heel.

Modifications

- Pad or donut the area during all activity as shown in **Figure 5-9**.
- Continue all non-weight-bearing activities such as swimming or biking.
- Continue all upper and lower extremity weight training.

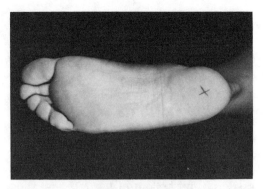

Figure 5-7. Location of heel bruise. Tender area is marked with an X.

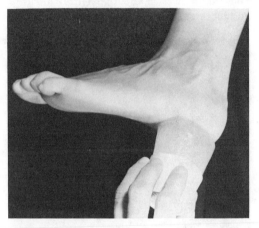

Figure 5-8. Ice cup applied to heel.

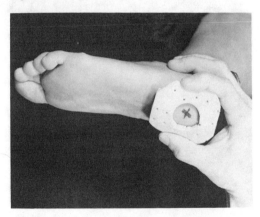

Figure 5-9. Donut pad used to take pressure off affected area during walking.

- Perform exercises 1, 2, 3, 4, 6, 7, and 8. These should be done without pain.

Pain on Bottom of Foot, Back Toward Heel
(Plantar Fasciitis, Bone Spurs, Heel Spurs)

Plantar fasciitis is an inflammation and/or a tearing of a broad band of connective tissue on the bottom of the foot that runs from the heel to the forefoot (plantar fascia). This connective tissue pulls from the heel and produces an irritation **(Figure 5-10)**. Re-peated irritation may cause the formation of a sharp boney growth in the area of the heel, known as a heel or bone spur **(Figure 5-11)**. It may also develop into a stress fracture in the heel if the pain is ignored.

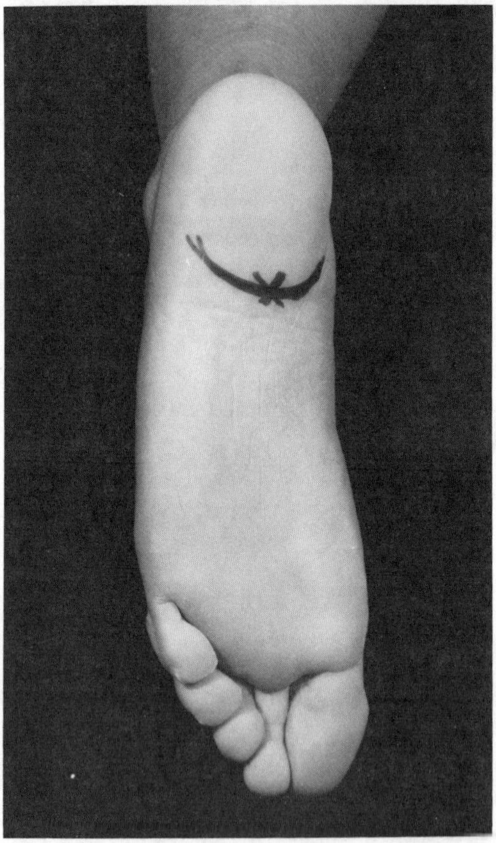

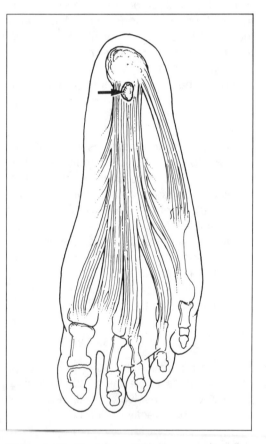

Figure 5-10. Common location of irritation of plantar fascia.

Figure 5-11. Heel or bone spur.

Symptoms

Pain is usually localized on the bottom of the foot toward the region of the heel, but not directly on the heel. Pain radiates toward the ball of the foot under the surface. There is increased pain with weight-bearing activities when there is extreme pressure on the arch. It is characteristic of this problem for pain to be more intense in the morning or after resting for an extended period. The pain will subside to a degree as weight bearing continues, but it will intensify with lengthy or excessive activity.

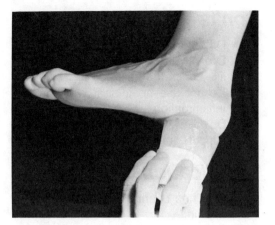

Figure 5-12. Ice cup applied to heel.

Do's

- Use rest, ice, compression, and elevation for 20 to 30 minutes after activity or excessive weight bearing.
- Use an ice cup **(Figure 5-12)**. Apply in small, circular motions until ice is gone. This may be used after activity or weight bearing as an alternative to ice, compression, and elevation.
- Utilize an arch taping **(Figure 5-13)**.
- Use soft orthotics.
- Pad or donut if pain is localized in a specific spot **(Figure 5-14)**.

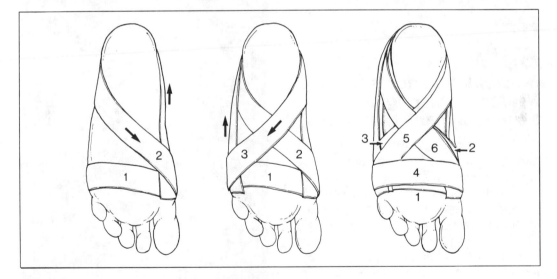

Figure 5-13. X-arch taping: Use 1-inch white adhesive tape.
    1. Place a strip around the ball of the foot.
    2. Start the next strip on the side of the foot beginning at the base of the big toe. Take tape around heel, crossing arch, returning to starting point.
    3. Third strip is same as 2nd strip, except that it is started on the little toe side of the foot.
    4. Lock each series by placing tape around ball of foot.
    5-6. A series of 3 X-strips is usually applied.

Don'ts

- Do not run on toes.
- Do not run or jump on hard surfaces like concrete or tile floors.
- Do not use heat, as it will increase inflammation.
- Do not walk in bare feet, as the lack of support puts more stress on the arch.

Modifications

- Continue bearing weight to the point of pain.
- Utilize arch taping or prescribed orthotics.
- Concentrate on a heel toe movement gait.
- Perform non-weight-bearing activities such as swimming or biking if pain is intense.
- Perform exercises 1, 2, 3, 6, 7, and 9. These should be done without pain.

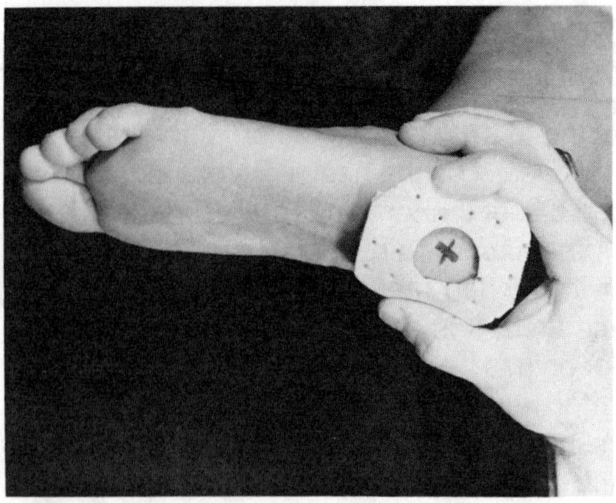

Figure 5-14. Donut pad to take pressure off affected area.

Sharp Pain in Ball of Foot, Between Toes
(Neuroma: Morton's Neuroma, Interdigital Neuroma, Plantar Neuroma)

A neuroma is a swelling of a portion of a nerve. In the foot it may be called a Morton's, interdigital, or plantar neuroma. It usually affects the nerve located between the 3rd and 4th toes or the 2nd and 3rd toes in the area of the ball of the foot **(Figure 5-15)**. The swelling (neuroma) occurs where branches of the nerve cross in an X-like pattern causing the enlargement of the nerve. A neuroma develops when the toes or the bones in the ball of the foot are pushed together, causing irritation to the nerve.

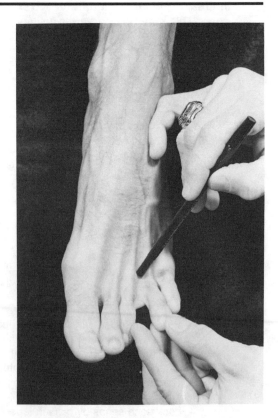

Figure 5-15. Common location of a neuroma.

Symptoms

Pain develops in the ball of the foot and creates a tingling, radiating sensation out to the end of the involved toes. The pain begins gradually but gets progressively worse. This condition is exacerbated by tight, narrow shoes. Pain increases during walking or physical activity associated with weight bearing and rotation on the balls of the foot. Descending stairs in soft shoes or no shoes aggravates the problem. There is soreness at the specific location of the nerve in the ball of the foot. This problem may be relieved by adjusting mechanics and/or footwear.

Do's

- Rest.
- Use ice, compression, and elevation for 20 to 30 minutes following activity or excessive weight-bearing (**Figure 5-16**).
- Use an ice cup (**Figure 5-17**).
- Wear wide shoes during normal weight bearing and activity.
- Use orthotics or arch supports.
- Pad the area below the metatarsal heads (**Figure 5-18**). This will eliminate direct pressure on the painful area.

Don'ts

- Do not wear tight, narrow shoes.
- Do not jump on the ball of the foot.
- Do not run or jump on hard surfaces.

Modifications

- Wear wide shoes at all times.
- Limit any activity that produces pain in the ball of the foot.
- Continue non-weight-bearing activities like swimming or biking.
- Stretch the forefoot and heel cords.
- Do exercises 5, 6, 7, 8, and 9. These should be done without pain.

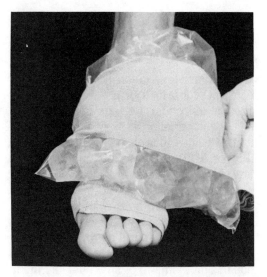

Figure 5-16. Ice, compression, and elevation of foot area.

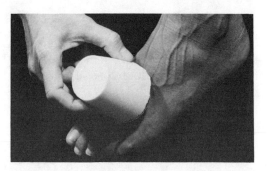

Figure 5-17. Applying ice cup to foot.

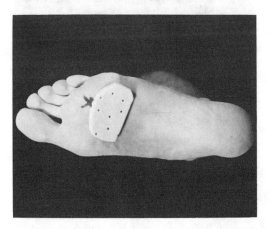

Figure 5-18. Pad to relieve pressure on affected area.

Curled-up Toes
(Hammer Toes, Claw Toes)

Hammer toes is the name for a condition where the toes or a toe are in a bent position, exposing the tops of the joints to friction and irritation as they come into contact with the underside surface of shoes **(Figure 5-19)**. The tendons under the toes are very tight; therefore, the toes cannot straighten or return to normal positions. Some persons are born with this problem, but it may be caused by wearing shoes which are too short and narrow over a long period of time. Unfortunately, once a person has this problem, he or she must tolerate it, use pads, or have it surgically corrected.

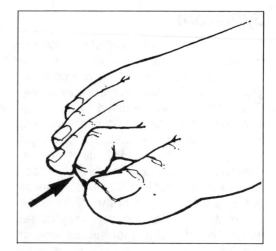

Figure 5-19. Curled-up toe.

Symptoms

The toes are visibly flexed. There is a callus formation on the top of the toes and discomfort due to the excessive friction and irritation.

Do's

- Wear shoes of proper length and width.
- Pad the top of the toe to reduce friction and irritation **(Figure 5-20)**.
- Maintain the normal range of motion of the toes by stretching the toes to avoid rigid positions and tightening of the tendons.

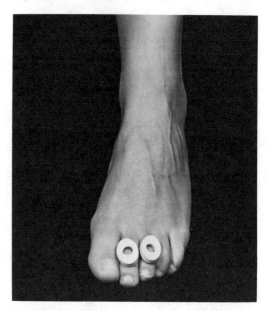

Figure 5-20. Donut pads on top of toes to reduce friction.

Don'ts

- Do not wear shoes that are too tight, narrow, or short.
- Do not wear shoes which rub excessively on the tops of the toes.
- Do not ignore this problem.

Modifications

- Maintain normal weight-bearing activities to the point of pain.
- Pad the tops of the toes to reduce irritation.
- Adjust the mechanics of walking and running to decrease symptoms.
- Do exercises 1 through 9. These should be done without pain.

Large Big Toe Joint
(Bunion-Hallus Valgus)

A bunion is an enlargement of the joint of the big toe. The joint is made more prominent by the big toe deviation toward the smaller toes **(Figure 5-21)**. An individual may be born with this, or it may develop over time if one wears shoes that are too tight, narrow, and pointed. The prominence on the inside of the foot at the location of the big toe becomes sore and irritated due to pressure from footwear. This condition may be relieved by adjusting foot mechanics, footwear, or both, but it may have to be surgically corrected if the symptoms are too painful.

Symptoms

The symptoms of a bunion include pain directly on the prominence with soreness in the big and/or 2nd toe. There will be increased pain if weight-bearing activities are increased or if tight shoes are worn. The deformity in this area may progress and move the big toe under the 2nd toe creating a hammer toe deformity.

Do's

- Wear wide shoes.
- Rest.
- Use ice, compression, and elevation after activity or excessive weight bearing to help realign joint.
- Use a toe spacer **(Figure 5-22)**.
- Pad the area directly over the bunion.

Don'ts

- Do not wear tight, pointed shoes.
- Do not utilize heat, as it will increase inflammation.
- Do not run or jump excessively on the balls of your feet.

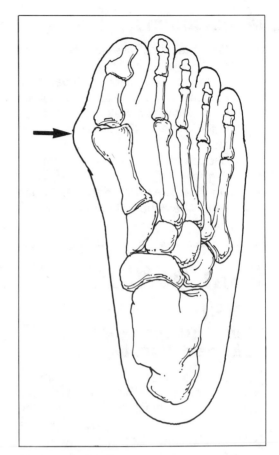

Figure 5-21. Bunion.

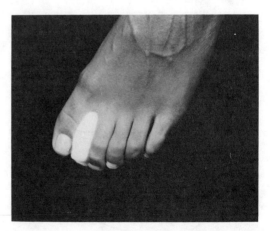

Figure 5-22. Toe spacer used to help relieve symptoms of a bunion.

Modifications

- Continue all activities as tolerated to the point of pain.
- Consider specialized footwear such as custom-made, extra wide shoes with expandable materials in the ball of the foot area to accommodate this problem.
- Use toe spacers between the 1st and 2nd toes.
- Do exercises 1 through 9. These should be done without pain.

Pain behind Heel
(Pump Bumps, Post-Calcaneal Bursitis)

Post-calcaneal bursitis is an inflammation of the pad-like sac (bursa) located at the back of the heel in the area where the Achilles tendon attaches to the heel **(Figure 5-23)**. It is a chronic condition frequently caused by pressure and rubbing of the upper edge of a shoe in the heel area of an adult. This produces tenderness and irritation. This problem may be relieved when the irritating factors are removed.

Symptoms

The symptoms of pump bumps are pain and irritation directly on the heel area in the location of the Achilles tendon attachment. Swelling is often present, and there is a specific spot on the heel where the pain is most intense.

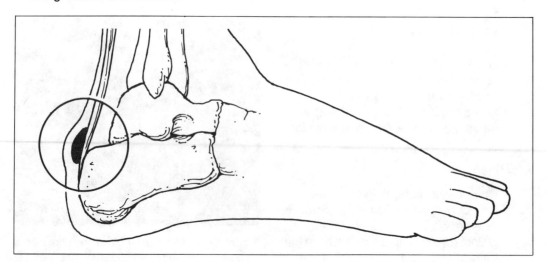

Figure 5-23. Location of "Pump Bumps" - inflamed bursa.

Do's

- Use an ice cup **(Figure 5-24)**. Apply in circular motions until ice is gone.
- Adjust or change shoes to eliminate the pressure of the back of the shoe on this area. High heels with rigid backs have to be changed or softened.
- Pad or donut the area to avoid pressure **(Figure 5-25)**.

Don'ts

- Don't wear high heels that cause direct pressure on the heel.
- Don't wear sport shoes with tabs that crease in this area.

Modifications

- Continue all activities as tolerated to the point of pain.
- Wear shoes with low heels and soft tabs.
- Do exercises 1, 2, 3, 6, and 7. These should be done without pain.

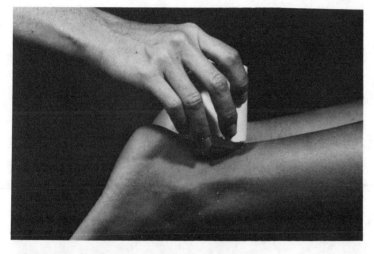

Figure 5-24. Applying an ice cup to affected area.

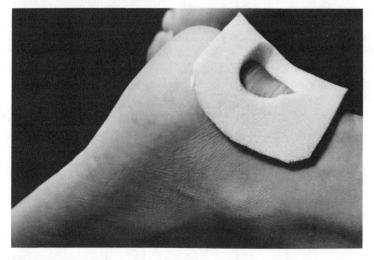

Figure 5-25. Donut pad to relieve pressure on affected area.

Pain in Heel of Child
(Severs Disease, Apophysitis of the Calcaneus)

Severs Disease occurs in physically active children between the ages of 8 and 13. It occurs at the top of the heel at the junction of the bottom and back **(Figure 5-26)**. The stress and tension of the heel cord puts pressure on the boney attachment and causes irritation at the point.

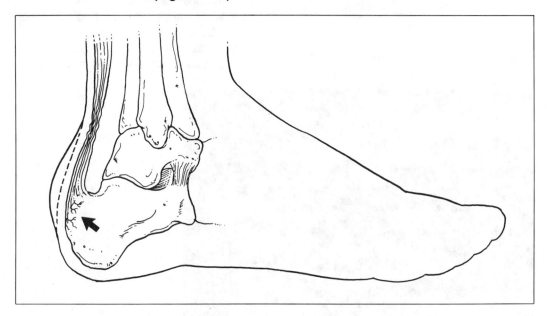

Figure 5-26. Location of Severs Disease.

Symptoms

There is pain and swelling at the back of the heel especially with running and exercising. Usually the problem is not caused by a specific injury. As an individual gets older and the bones harden, the condition will subside.

Do's

- Rest.
- Use ice, compression, and elevation.

Don'ts

- Do not do any heel cord stretching.
- Do not stretch the foot upward toward shin.

Modifications

- Elevate both heels by wearing one-fourth inch heel lifts.

Plantar Wart

A plantar wart is a wart found on the sole of the foot **(Figure 5-27)**. It is caused by a virus infection. Many people confuse a plantar wart with a callus. Plantar warts occur anywhere on the sole of the foot, whereas calluses occur only on pressure points. A plantar wart has a distinct edge with a central core. It does not project beyond the skin surface, and sometimes appears to be growing inward. There is excessive thickening of the skin. There may be several plantar warts in one area forming a satellite configuration.

Symptoms

There is localized pain during weight-bearing activities, specifically in the area of the plantar wart. It may feel like you are stepping on broken glass. The wart will appear as a small black dot in a center surrounded by a clearer callus area.

Do's

- Donut or pad area to take direct pressure off wart **(Figure 5-28)**.
- Keep callus build-up around wart (not the wart itself) filed down.
- Do exercises 1 through 9. These should be done without pain.

Don'ts

- Don't try to file away the wart, as this will cause irritation and possible infection.

Modifications

- See a podiatrist or a physician for options for care or removal.

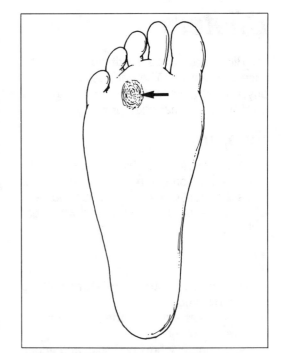

Figure 5-27. Plantar wart.

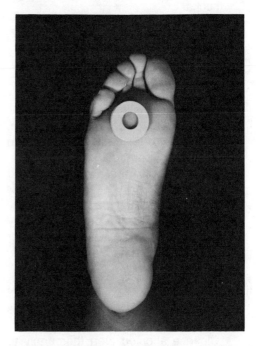

Figure 5-28. Donut pad to take pressure off plantar wart.

Blisters

Blisters are areas of irritation caused by excessive friction. They are common in all physical activity and can become extremely disabling if not managed properly.

Symptoms

The symptoms of blisters are specific areas of irritation **(Figure 5-29)**. In the foot these are usually found on the ball, the heel, or both. The blister may be filled with clear or bloody fluid.

Do's

- Reduce friction—blisters will be prevented.
- Use vaseline or lubricate common areas of friction.
- Eliminate seams on socks and ridges on the inside of shoes, or wear tube socks.
- Wear two pairs of socks.
- Break in new shoes gradually.

Don'ts

- Do not go sockless.
- Do not allow callus build-up to form— use a callus file or pumice stone. (Blisters under calluses are much more difficult to treat.)
- Do not apply heat to the affected area.
- Do not puncture blister—you may cause infection. If it opens, cut away the dead skin that was over the blister and keep the area clean and dry.

Modifications

- Continue all weight-bearing activities to the point of pain.
- Cleanse affected area thoroughly to prevent infection.
- Use donut pad to reduce pressure on affected area **(Figure 5-30)**.
- Cover with sterile dressing when you are not active.

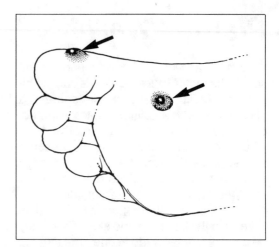

Figure 5-29. Blisters.

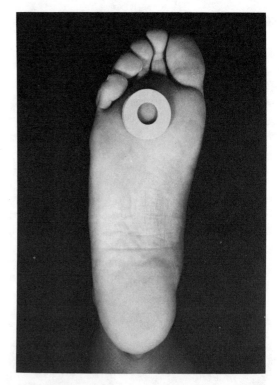

Figure 5-30. Donut pad to relieve pressure on blister.

- If the blister skin comes loose or is broken open, remove the dead skin and keep the area clean until new, thick skin develops.
- Be aware of signs of infection (swelling, radiating red streaks), and see a physician immediately if these occur.

Foot Exercises

The following exercises should be used with the problems described in this chapter. They are designed to restrengthen the musculature that surrounds the injured area to hasten recovery and ensure a safe return to activity. They will also help prevent injuries or injury recurrences. The exercises can be done anywhere, and no special equipment is needed. These exercises should be performed *without pain*, twice a day, as long as the problem is present.

1. Toe Grip and Spread

Sitting or standing, curl the toes on one foot as tightly as possible **(Figure 5-31)**; then spread your toes as widely as possible **(Figure 5-32)**. Do this 15 to 30 times with each foot, twice a day.

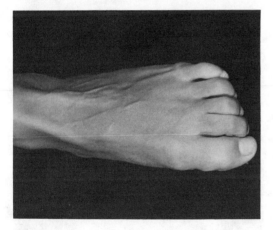

Figure 5-31.

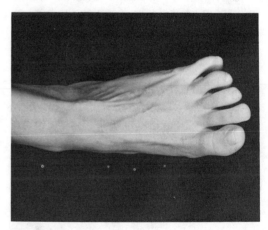

Figure 5-32.

2. Marble Pick-Up

Sitting or standing, pick up marbles or small wads of paper with the toes on your injured foot and place them in a cup or container **(Figure 5-33)**. Do this approximately 20 times, twice a day.

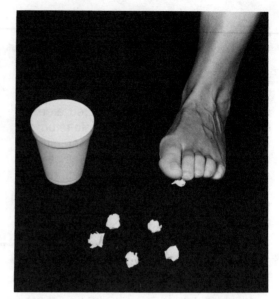

Figure 5-33.

3. Towel Pull

Sitting in a chair, place a towel flat on the floor in front of you. Keeping the heel of your injured foot on the floor, use your toes to pull the towel toward you **(Figure 5-34)**. When the entire towel is in front of you, straighten it out and repeat. Do this 10 times, twice a day. To make this exercise more difficult, add a weight or large book on the towel for resistance **(Figure 5-35)**.

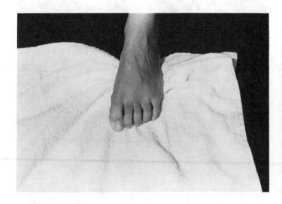

Figure 5-34.

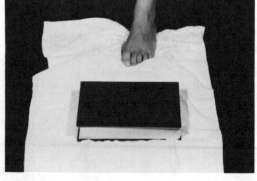

Figure 5-35.

4. Heel Raises

a. Stand with feet flat on the floor and arms down at your side. Raise heels and slowly go up on toes. Do this with feet in 3 positions. 1. Toes pointed straight ahead **(Figure 5-36)**. 2. Toes pointed in **(Figure 5-37)**. 3. Toes pointed out **(Figure 5-38)**. Repeat 10 to 20 times, twice a day.

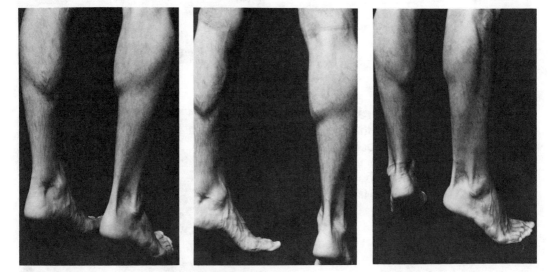

Figure 5-36.   Figure 5-37.   Figure 5-38.

b. Stand on a step, heels off the back edge, with hands on hips or out straight in front **(Figure 5-39)**. Drop heels below step **(Figure 5-40)**, slowly raise heels and go up on toes **(Figure 5-41)**, and slowly lower. Repeat 10 to 20 times, twice a day.

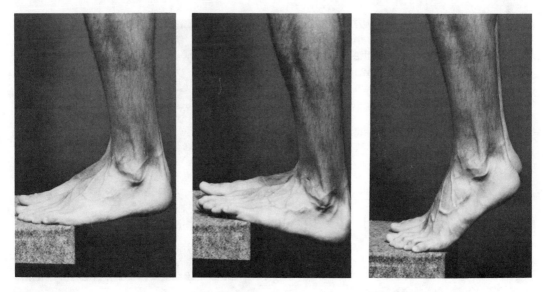

Figure 5-39.   Figure 5-40.   Figure 5-41.

5. *Toe Raises*

Stand with feet flat on the floor hands at side. Raise your toes and the front of your feet off the floor **(Figure 5-42)**. Repeat 10 to 20 times, twice a day.

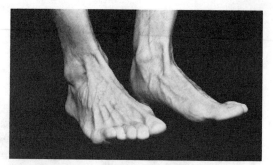

Figure 5-42.

6. *Inward Motion (Inversion)*

Sit or stand with heels on the floor, arms at side. Move the injured foot off the floor and inward toward other foot **(Figure 5-43** — shown with rubber tubing resistance.) Repeat 10 to 20 times, twice a day.

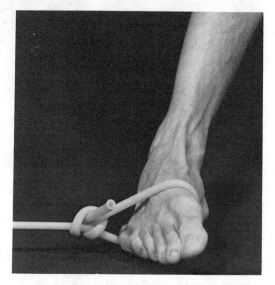

Figure 5-43.

7. *Outward Motion (Eversion)*

Sit or stand with heels on the floor arms at side. Move forefoot of the injured foot off floor and outward, away from your foot **(Figure 5-44** — shown with rubber tubing resistance.) Repeat 10 to 20 times, twice a day.

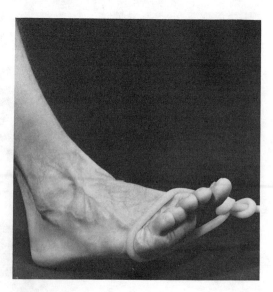

Figure 5-44.

8. Heel Cord/Calf Stretch

Stand with feet flat on floor, heels down. One leg should be bent forward, with the back leg straight and both heels flat. Lean forward, shifting weight to front leg, keeping the back leg straight **(Figure 5-45)**. Do not lift heels off the floor. Hold for 8 to 10 seconds, change legs, and repeat. Do 5 to 8 times with each leg twice a day. (Stretch should be felt in the belly of the muscle, *not* in the tendons behind the joint.)

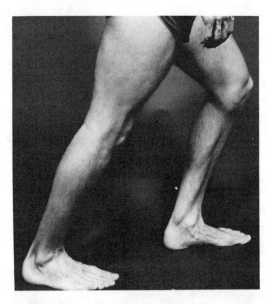

Figure 5-45.

9. Soleus Stretch

Stand with feet flat on floor, heels down. One leg should be bent forward, with the back leg's knee slightly bent and the heels *flat* **(Figure 5-46)**. Lean forward, shifting weight to the front leg, keeping the back leg slightly flexed. Hold for 8 to 10 seconds, change legs and repeat. Do 5 to 8 times with each leg, twice daily. (Stretch should be felt in the belly of the muscle, not in the tendons behind the joint.)

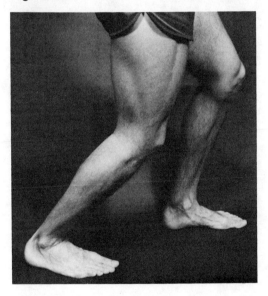

Figure 5-46.

The Ankle

Injuries to the ankle are extremely common during physical activity. Even though the ankle is structurally quite strong due to the arrangement of the bones, ligaments and muscles, it still is frequently injured. The most common injury is a sprained ankle.

Chapter **6**

Outer Ankle Sprain

A sprained ankle is usually a tear of the anterior talofibular ligament located just in front of the small ankle bone on the outside of the ankle **(Figure 6-1)**. You can normally treat this sprain yourself. Other ligaments around the ankle, especially on the other side, can be sprained. These are more serious injuries that require medical attention.

Any injury to the ligament or bones on the inner side of the ankle usually represents a serious problem and requires a physician's evaluation. Ankle sprains most frequently occur when the foot turns inward and stress is placed on the outside of the ankle **(Figure 6-2)**. Refer to Chapter 1 for an explanation of the degrees of sprains.

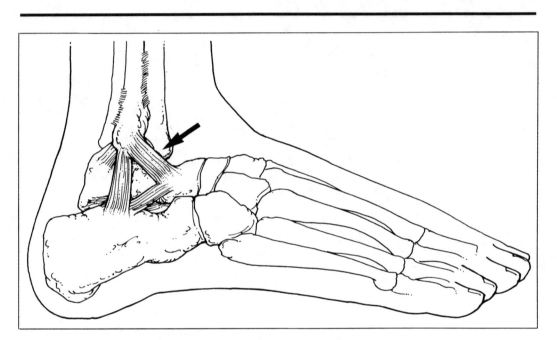

Figure 6-1. Frequently torn ligament in the ankle—anterior talofibular.

Symptoms

There is a specific area of pain (point tenderness) directly over the injured ligament. Swelling takes place right in the area of the injury, and within a day the swelling can spread throughout the entire ankle joint, involving both sides. It is important to pinpoint the exact location of pain immediately after injury. As the ankle swells and becomes more inflammed, it is much more difficult to determine the location and severity of the problem. The amount of swelling and pain do not necessarily indicate the degree of the injury. Individuals swell differently and have different levels of pain tolerance. The location is most important.

The injured area can also become black and blue, and signs of bruising may be seen throughout the entire foot and ankle.

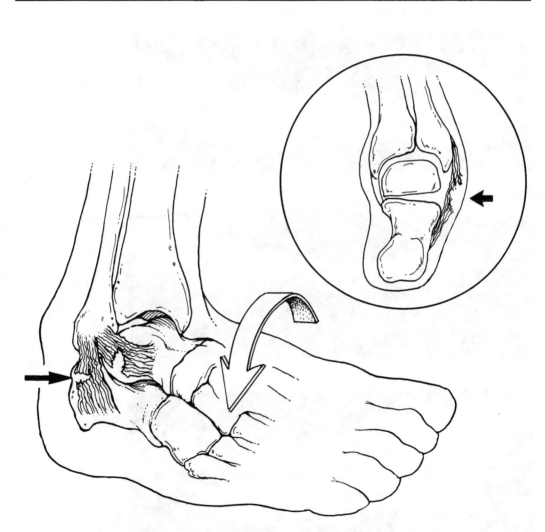

Figure 6-2. Inward motion of foot and ankle, which commonly causes sprains. Inset shows view of sprained ligament from behind ankle.

Do's

- Rest.
- Use compression, ice, and elevation **(Figures 6-3, 4, and 5)**.
- Apply compression with horseshoe pad to force swelling away from ankle bone and help to maintain better joint motion **(Figure 6-6)**.
- Apply adhesive tape once swelling is controlled, as illustrated **(Figure 6-7)**.
- Use crutches if walking is painful or extremely impaired.
- See a physician if tenderness is anywhere other than in the anterior talofibular ligament.

Don'ts

- Do not use heat at any time.
- Do not do any inward movements with the foot and ankle that could stress the injured ligament.
- Do not jump or twist, since the ankle is unstable and further damage could occur.

Figure 6-3 to 5. Compression, ice, and elevation of ankle.

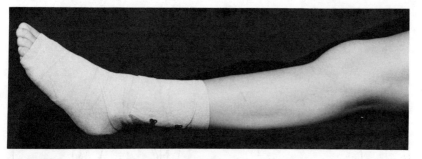

Figure 6-3.

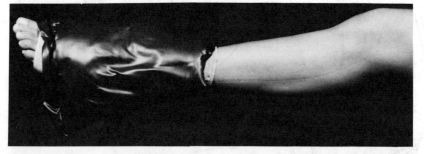

Figure 6-4.

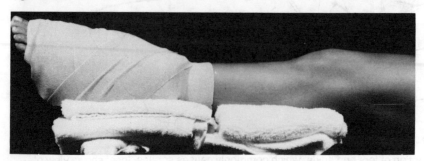

Figure 6-5.

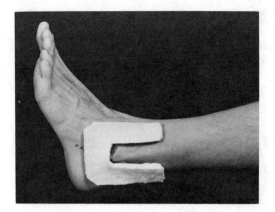

Figure 6-6. Horseshoe pad to reduce swelling.

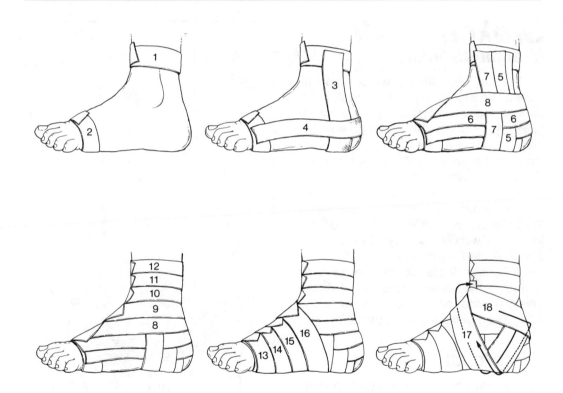

Figure 6-7. Adhesive tape support for ankle: Use 1½ inch white adhesive tape.
    1. Place one anchor strip around top of ankle.
    2. Place one anchor strip around foot.
    3. Run vertical strip from inside of ankle, under heel, to top of anchor on outside of ankle.
    4. Run horizontal strip from inside of foot, around heel, to anchor around foot.
    5-8. Repeat vertical and horizontal strips two more times.
    9-12. Close off upper ankle with separate circular strips.
    13-16. Close off lower foot with separate circular strips.
    17-18. Apply figure 8 and heel locks to ensure stability.

Modifications

- Perform non-weight-bearing exercises like biking and weight training.
- Do exercises 1 and 5, without pain.
- Use a brace support **(Figure 6-8)**.
- Apply tape support illustrated in **(Figure 6-7)**.

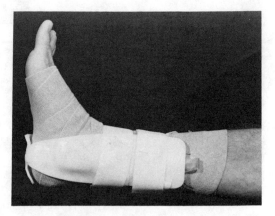

Figure 6-8. Brace support for ankle.

Broken Ankle
(Fractured Ankle)

Fractures are almost as common as sprains. Severe pain, inability to walk, a deformity, or any combination of these symptoms may help you with the diagnosis. The area of tenderness will be on a bone, not in the area of a ligament. Many times it is difficult to tell whether an ankle is just sprained or broken since the symptoms for both problems are similar. Occasionally a bone inside the ankle can break. Obviously it is difficult to be sure without an x-ray. Have a physician evaluate the problem.

A bone in the ankle can be fractured whenever the ankle is forcefully twisted. This may occur on the inside (tibia) or outside (fibula) of the ankle **(Figure 6-9)**.

Symptoms

There will be a distinct area of pain directly over a bone in the ankle. Swelling will be present. Discoloration may be noticeable. Movement of the ankle will be limited. It may be painful to put weight on the injured ankle. This injury is caused by a specific event. At the time of incident, you may have felt a sharp, electric shock-like pain in the ankle followed by immediate numbness.

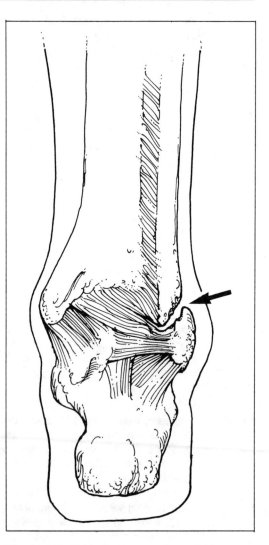

Figure 6-9. Ankle fracture on the outside.

Do's

- Rest.
- Use, ice, compression, elevation, as in **Figure 6-3**.
- Get an x-ray.

Don'ts

- Do not walk or put weight on the injured ankle.

Modifications

- Use crutches if walking is painful.
- Keep ankle supported in a brace and a wrap, as in **Figure 6-8**.

Ankle Exercises

The following exercises should be used with the previous problems. They are designed to restrengthen the musculature that surrounds the injured area to hasten recovery and ensure a safe return to activity. They will also help prevent injuries or injury recurrences. Following any injury, they should be started as soon as they can be performed correctly, without pain. Pain should never be present during these exercises at any time.

The exercises can be done anywhere, and no special equipment is needed. These exercises should be performed 2 to 3 times a day, as long as the problem is present.

1. Alphabet Writing (Increases Motion in Joint)

Sit with the foot and the heel of your injured ankle suspended. Make capital letters of the alphabet with your foot, with toes pointed. Do the entire alphabet 3 times, twice daily (**Figure 6-10**).

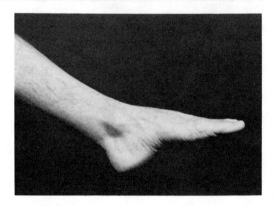

Figure 6-10.

2. Toe Grip and Spread

Sitting or standing, curl the toes on one foot as tightly as possible; then spread as widely as possible (**Figure 6-11 and 12**). Do this 15 to 30 times with each foot, twice a day.

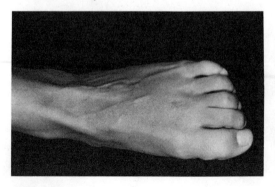

Figure 6-11.

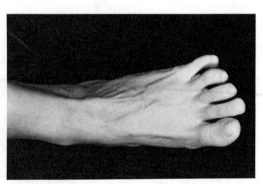

Figure 6-12.

3. Heel Raises

a. Stand with feet flat on floor, arms down at side. Raise heels and slowly go up on toes. Do this with feet in 3 positions: 1. Toes pointed straight ahead **(Figure 6-13)**. 2. Toes pointed in **(Figure 6-14)**. 3. Toes pointed out **(Figure 6-15)**. Repeat 10 to 20 times, twice a day.

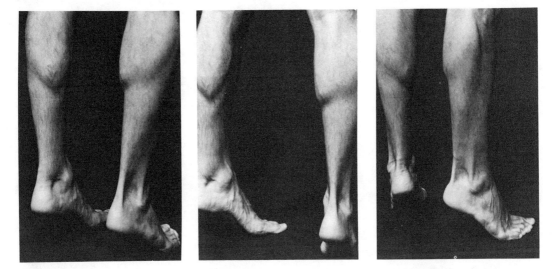

Figure 6-13.   Figure 6-14.   Figure 6-15.

b. Stand on a step with heels off back edge, hands on hips or straight out in front **(Figure 6-16)**. Drop heels below step **(Figure 6-17)**, slowly raise heels and go up on toes **(Figure 6-18)**, then slowly lower. Repeat 10 to 20 times, twice a day.

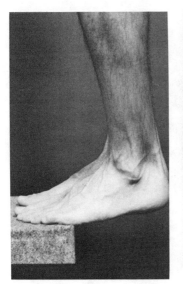 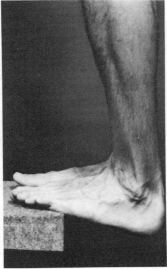 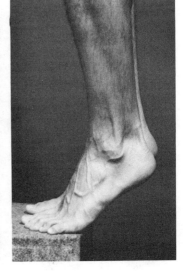

Figure 6-16.   Figure 6-17.   Figure 6-18.

4. Towel Pull

Sitting in a chair, place a towel flat on the floor in front of you. Keeping the heel of your injured ankle on the floor, use your toes to pull the towel toward you **(Figure 6-19)**. When the entire towel has been moved, straighten it out and repeat. Do this completely 5 to 10 times, twice a day. To make this exercise more difficult, add a weight or large book on the towel for resistance **(Figure 6-20)**.

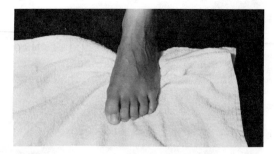

Figure 6-19.

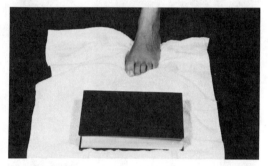

Figure 6-20.

5. Resistance Exercises With Tubing

Sit and attach one end of rubber tubing around a stationary object like a heavy chair or table. Attach other end around your injured foot. Pull foot against resistance of tubing out, in, up, and down **(Figure 6-21 and 22)**. Do 10 to 15 times, each way, twice daily.

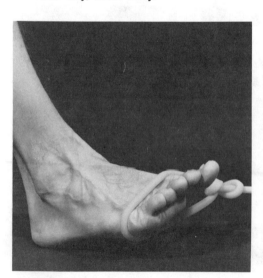

Figure 6-21.

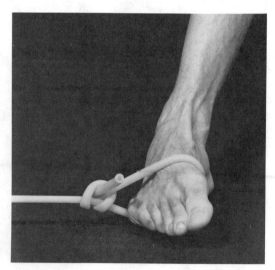

Figure 6-22.

The Lower Leg

The part of the lower body between the knee and ankle is called the lower leg. It is made up of 2 bones (the tibia and fibula), soft tissue, and muscle **(Figure 7-1)**. Because it helps to support the body during movement, the lower leg is subject to various stresses that may produce injury.

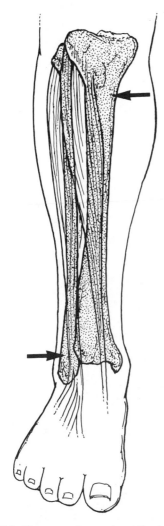

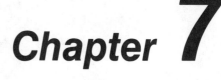

Figure 7-1. Bones and muscle of the lower leg; lower-fibula, upper-tibia.

Chapter **7**

Pain/Ache On Front Of Lower Leg
(Shin Splints)

Shin splints is a general term for any pain or discomfort located in the front or the side of the lower leg. This is usually over the tibia, which is the larger of the 2 lower leg bones **(Figure 7-2)**. Shin splints is a form of a stress fracture, described in Chapters 1 and 5. The damage to the tibia produces muscle inflammation. Do not "run through" this problem, as it will get worse. Various factors may cause shin splints, including poor shoes, sudden change in training habits, incorrect running mechanics, or overtraining. You must try to determine what caused your particular injury so you can correct the problem and prevent recurrences.

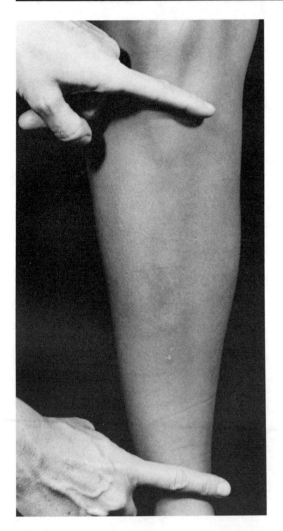

Figure 7-2. Common location of shin splints, over the tibia.

Symptoms

Shin splints are characterized by pain in the shin area on one or both legs. As you touch the affected area, you may find local tenderness on the bone. Pain and aching in the front of the lower leg will be felt after activity and sometimes even during activity.

Do's

- Rest. Adjust or lessen your activity training level.
- Use ice, compression, and elevation.
- Apply an ice cup **(Figure 7-3)**.
- Use X-arch taping to support arches **(Figure 7-4)**.
- Use orthotic inserts for shoes.

Don'ts

- Do not ignore this problem, as it will get worse.
- Do not continue activities that cause pain or discomfort in the affected area.

Modifications

- Continue non-weight-bearing activities such as swimming, biking, and weight lifting.
- Do exercises 1 through 8, without pain.
- Determine what has caused your problem and correct and/or modify it.

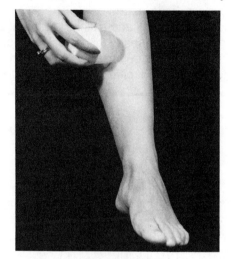

Figure 7-3. Ice cup applied to shin.

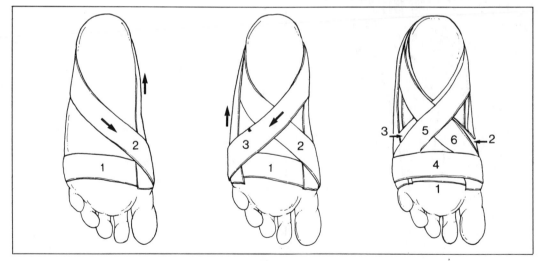

Figure 7-4. X-arch taping: Use 1-inch white adhesive tape.
1. Place a strip around the ball of the foot.
2. Start the next strip on the side of the foot beginning at the base of the big toe. Take tape around heel, crossing arch, returning to starting point.
3. Third strip is same as 2nd strip, except that it is started on the little toe side of the foot.
4. Lock each series by placing tape around ball of foot.
5-6. A series of 3 X-strips is usually applied.

Calf or Heel Pain
(Achilles Tendon Rupture, Achilles Tendinitis, Soleus-Gastrocnemius Rupture, Plantaris Rupture)

The large muscle in the back of your calf (the gastrocnemius) runs from slightly above the knee, narrows into the Achilles tendon (heel cord), and attaches to the heel **(Figure 7-5)**. Injuries to this muscle can occur throughout its entire length. You need to determine the specific location of tender-ness before you can identify your injury. You should touch and push in on the affected area to determine the location of pain.

If tenderness is located down towards the heel in the area of the heel cord, the Achilles tendon may be inflammed (Achilles tendinitis) or torn (Achilles tendon rupture) **(Figure 7-6)**. If the pain is higher up within the muscle mass, one of the calf muscles (soleus, gastrocnemius, or plantaris) may be torn **(Figure 7-7)**.

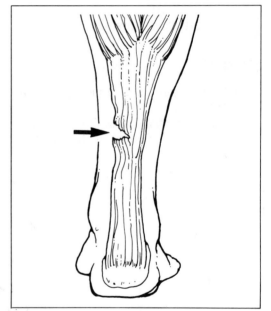

Figure 7-6. Tenderness in heel area (Achilles tendon).

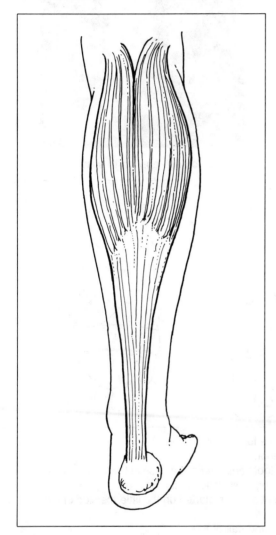

Figure 7-5. Calf muscle (gastrocnemius).

Symptoms

If the Achilles tendon or a calf muscle is completely torn, you will not be able to walk without crutches. You may be able to move your foot up and down when sitting, but not when standing or walking. There will be specific pain and possibly some swelling in the area of the tear. You may have heard a sudden "snap" or "pop" at the time of the injury.

To determine if the Achilles tendon is ruptured, do the Thompson Test by kneeling on a chair with your feet extended over the edge. Squeeze the calf muscle of the injured leg. Watch to see if the foot moves **(Figure 7-8)**. If the foot does *not* move, the tendon may be ruptured and you should see a physician immediately.

The symptoms of Achilles tendinitis are tenderness to the touch and pain with activity. There may be some discomfort and stiffness in the tendon area when you move your foot up and down. This is a chronic overuse problem which comes on gradually.

If the tenderness is up in the muscle area and you can still walk, some muscle fibers may have been strained, but not totally torn. This usually is a 1st or 2nd degree strain. There will be stiffness and tightness in the affected muscle. You will be able to perform most activities, but pain will remind you that there is an injured area in your muscle.

For severe muscle strains and ruptures, you will remember a specific incident that caused the pain or injury. If you cannot recall a specific event, then the problem is less severe.

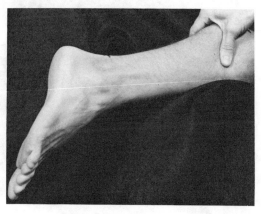

Figure 7-8. Thompson Test for torn Achilles tendon.

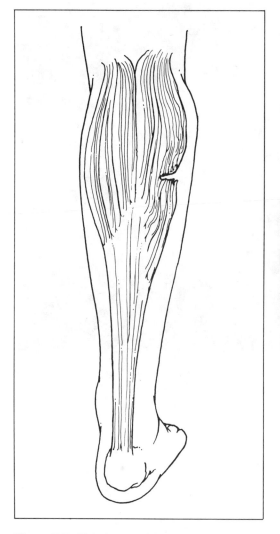

Figure 7-7. Pain in muscle mass.

Do's

- Use rest, ice, compression, and elevation.
- Use crutches if walking is painful.
- Put heel pad in shoes to take stress off calf and the heel cord. Place in both shoes to keep leg lengths equal **(Figure 7-9)**.
- Recognize such signs of severity as: increasing pain with activity, inability to walk, and extreme tenderness.

Don'ts

- Do not ignore these problems.
- Do not continue exercises that cause pain in the affected area.

Modifications

- Do non-weight-bearing exercises such as swimming, bicycling, and weight training.
- Do exercises 3, 4, 7, and 8 without pain. These exercises are *not* appropriate if a rupture has occurred.

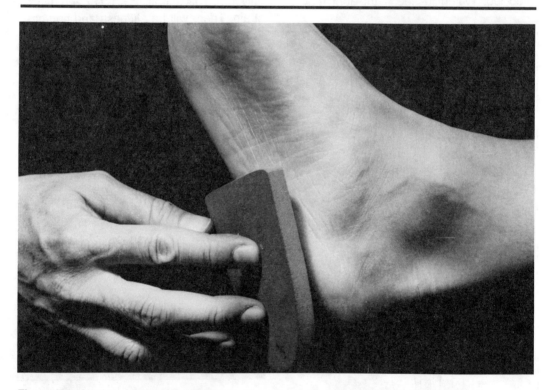

Figure 7-9. Heel pad (placed in both shoes) to relieve stress on heel cord and calf muscle.

Cramp in Back Of Lower Leg

(Calf Cramp, Leg Muscle Spasm)

A common location of muscle cramps is the calf. The causes of calf muscle cramps include fatigue, excessive activity, and loss of fluids. Calf cramps are impossible to predict and may occur during activity or even when you are asleep.

Symptoms

Calf cramps produce extreme pain and discomfort in the affected muscle. The muscle remains tight and contracted. Some types may relax momentarily, but then return to a tightened state. Pain may radiate down the entire length of the muscle. It is very difficult to move the foot on the affected leg.

Do's

- Stand up and stretch your heel cord.
- Try to relax the affected leg.
- Apply firm hand pressure to affected muscle area.
- Pull feet up so the calf is stretched.

Don'ts

- Do not *vigorously* massage affected area. This may cause more cramping.
- Do not "run it off."

Modifications

- Stretch the muscle by raising your toes and foot toward the shin and holding for approximately 8 seconds. Slowly release, and repeat until relief is felt **(Figure 7-10)**.
- If cramps recur, make sure that your diet contains the right minerals (salt, potassium, and calcium) and enough water to provide for normal muscle function.

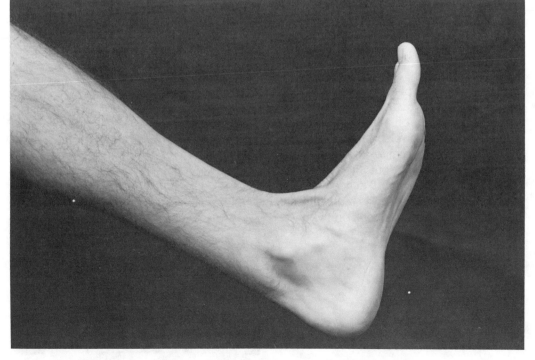

Figure 7-10. Moving toes and foot toward shin to help relieve cramp in calf.

Lower Leg Exercises

The following exercises should be used with the previous problems. They are designed to restrengthen the musculature that surrounds the injured area to hasten recovery and ensure a safe return to activity. They will also help prevent injuries or injury recurrences. Following any injury, they should be started as soon as they can be performed correctly, without pain. Pain should never be present during these exercises at any time. The exercises can be done anywhere, and no special equipment is needed. These exercises should be performed 2 to 3 times a day, as long as the problem is present.

1. Toe Grip and Spread

Sitting or standing, curl the toes on one leg as tightly as possible, then spread them as widely as possible **(Figure 7-11 and 12)**. Do this 15 to 30 times with each foot, twice a day.

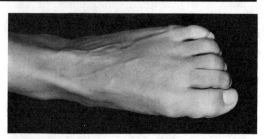

Figure 7-11.

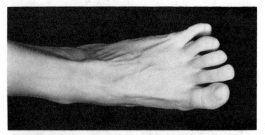

Figure 7-12.

2. Towel Pull

Sitting in a chair, place a towel flat on the floor in front of you. Keeping the heel of your injured leg on the floor, use your toes to pull the towel toward you **(Figure 7-13)**. When the entire towel has been moved, straighten it out and repeat. Do this completely 5 to 10 times, twice a day. To make this exercise more difficult, add a weight or large book on the towel to add resistance **(Figure 7-14)**.

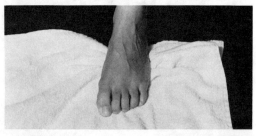

Figure 7-13.

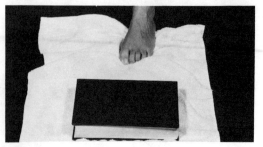

Figure 7-14.

3. Heel Raises

a. Stand with feet flat on floor, arms down at side. Raise heels and slowly go up on toes. Do this with feet in 3 positions: 1. Toes pointed straight ahead **(Figure 7-15)**. 2. Toes pointed in **(Figure 7-16)**. 3. Toes pointed out **(Figure 7-17)**. Repeat 10 to 20 times, twice daily.

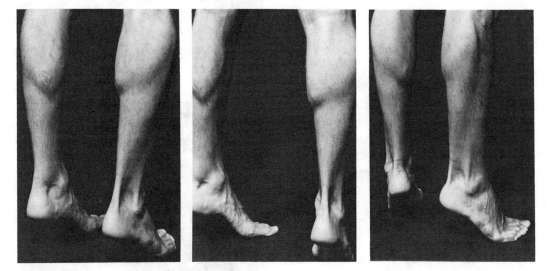

Figure 7-15.   Figure 7-16.   Figure 7-17.

b. Stand on a step with heel off back edge, with hands on hips or out straight in front **(Figure 7-18)**. Drop heels below step **(Figure 7-19)**, slowly raise heels and go up on toes **(Figure 7-20)**, and slowly lower. Repeat 10 to 20 times, twice daily.

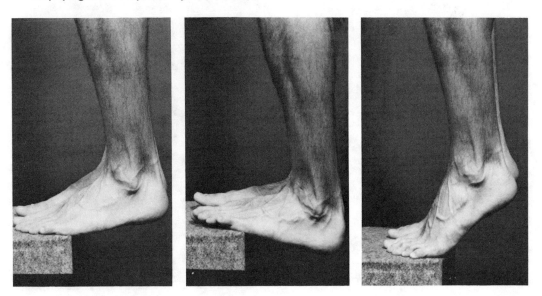

Figure 7-18.   Figure 7-19.   Figure 7-20.

4. *Toe Raises*

Stand with feet flat on the floor, hands at side. Raise your toes and the front of your feet off floor **(Figure 7-21)**. Repeat 10 to 20 times, twice a day.

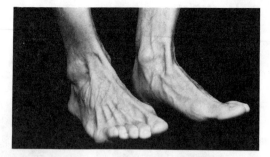

Figure 7-21.

5. *Inward Motion (Inversion)*

Sit or stand with heels on the floor, arms at side. Move forefoot of injured foot off the floor and inward, toward your other foot **(Figure 7-22)**. Repeat 10 to 20 times, twice daily.

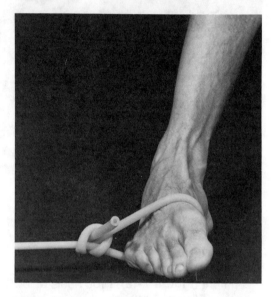

Figure 7-22.

6. *Outward Motion (Eversion)*

Sit or stand with heels on floor, arms at side. Move forefoot of injured foot off the floor and outward, away from your other foot **(Figure 7-23)**. Repeat 10 to 20 times, twice daily.

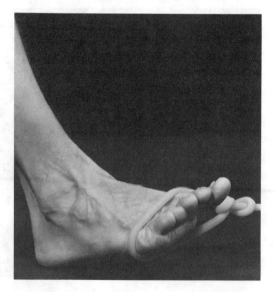

Figure 7-23.

7. *Heel Cord/Calf Stretch*

Stand with feet flat on floor, heels down. One leg should be bent forward, with the back leg straight. Lean forward, shifting weight to the front leg, keeping the back leg straight and both heels flat **(Figure 7-24)**. Hold for 8 to 10 seconds, change legs, and repeat. Do 5 to 8 times with each leg, twice a day. (Stretch should be felt in the belly of the muscle of the straightened back leg, *not* in the tendons behind the joint.)

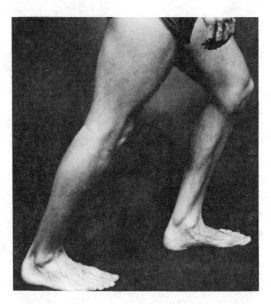

Figure 7-24

8. *Soleus Stretch*

Stand with feet flat on floor, heels down. One leg should be bent forward, with the back leg's knee slightly bent and both heels flat **(Figure 7-25)**. Lean forward, shifting weight to the front leg, keeping the back leg slightly flexed. Hold for 8 to 10 seconds, change legs and repeat. Do 5 to 8 times with each leg, twice daily. (Stretch should be felt in the belly of the muscle, not in the tendons behind the joint.)

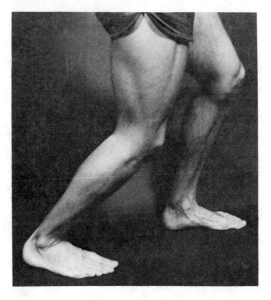

Figure 7-25.

The Knee

Injuries to the knee are very frightening. When you suffer a knee injury, you tend to think about all the athletes who ended their careers because of knee injuries. A knee injury *does not* have to mean the end of your activities. If treated properly, the majority of knee injuries heal as well as injuries in any other part of the body.

The knee is a complicated joint. Most physical activities place tremendous stress on the knees and their supporting structures. The knee is supported by a series of bands of tissue which hold one end of the upper leg bone (femur) to one end of the lower leg bones (tibia and fibula) **(Figure 8-1)**. These bands of tissue are called ligaments.

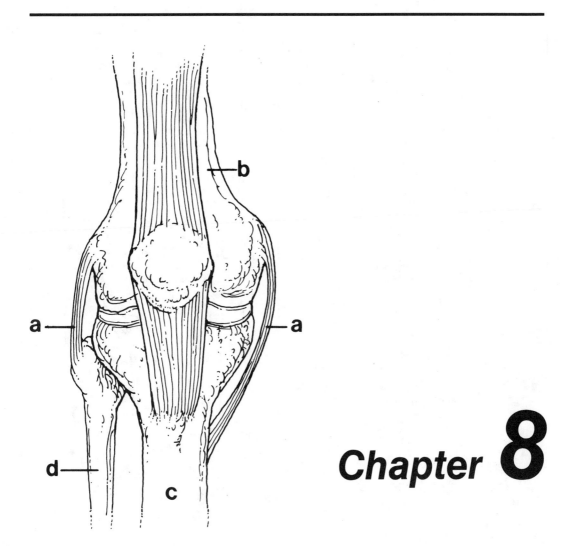

Chapter **8**

Figure 8-1. Knee joint; a) ligaments, b) femur, c) tibia, d) fibula.

Ligaments can become stretched or torn (sprained—see Chapter 1) when extreme stress is placed on them. When this occurs, the joint they support becomes unstable. There are ligaments on the inside and outside and in the middle of the knee **(Figure 8-2)**.

A piece of cartilage called the meniscus separates the femur from the tibia within the knee. There are 2 menisci in every knee **(Figure 8-3)**. This gristle-like substance lines the top surface of the tibia. It cushions the area where the femur sits on the tibia.

In determining what type of knee injury you have, it is important to determine where the tenderness is located. Pain may move throughout the joint, but specific areas of tenderness will lead you to the problem. For most knee injuries, you will remember an incident that caused pain and/or harm.

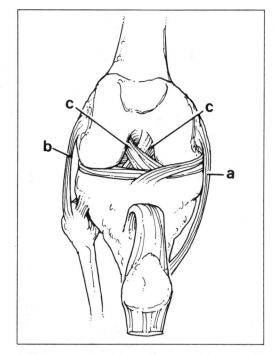

Figure 8-2. Knee ligaments on a) inside, b) outside, and c) in middle of knee.

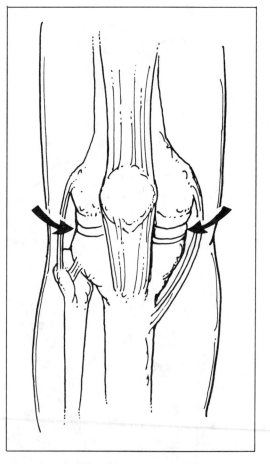

Figure 8-3. Knee cartilage (menisci).

Pain Inside Knee
(Medial Collateral Ligament Sprain)
Pain Outside Knee
(Lateral Collateral Ligament Sprain)

The ligaments on the inside and outside of the knee cross the joint and keep femur and tibia and fibula together **(Figure 8-4)**.

An injury to these ligaments may be minor (1st degree stretching or minor tear of the ligament—**Figure 8-5**), moderate (2nd degree or moderate tear of the ligament—**Figure 8-6**), or severe (3rd degree or total tear of the ligament—**Figure 8-7**).

The more severe the tear, the more unstable the joint becomes. Isolate the injury by feeling for specific tenderness. Also note if the knee feels loose and unstable, as if it could move in a direction it should not.

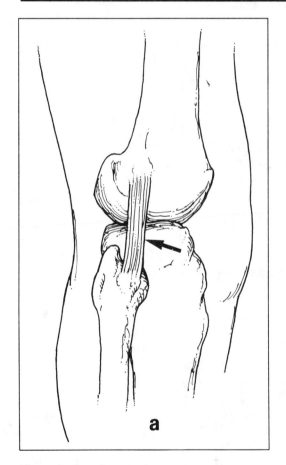

a

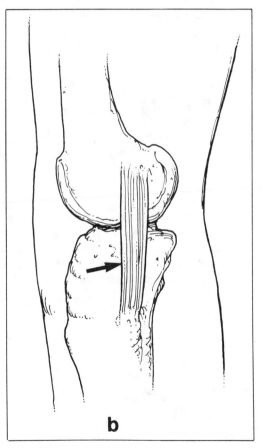

b

Figure 8-4. a. Outside (lateral) knee ligament
b. Inside (medial) knee ligament.

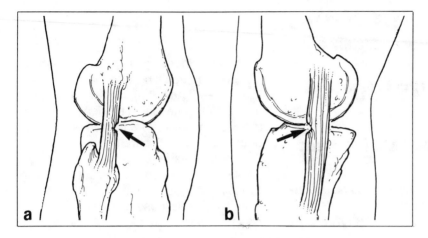

Figure 8-5. Minor, 1st degree tear of the: a. outside (lateral) knee ligament, b. inside (medial) knee ligament.

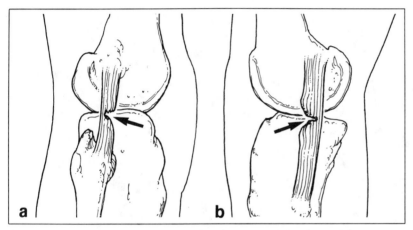

Figure 8-6. Moderate, 2nd degree tear of the: a. outside (lateral) knee ligament b. inside (medial) knee ligament.

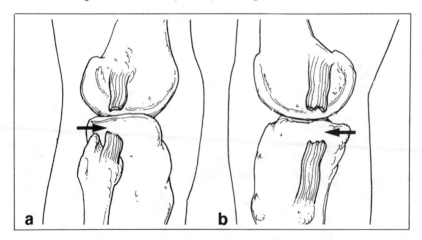

Figure 8-7. Severe, 3rd degree tear of the: a. outside (lateral) knee ligament b. inside (medial) knee ligament.

Symptoms

When a ligament is stretched and/or torn, there is pain, tenderness, and swelling. There are varying degrees of looseness or instability, and you may have trouble walking without crutches or a splint. There is a specific area of pain directly over the injured ligament or over the bone where it attaches **(Figure 8-8)**. You will remember a specific incident that caused the pain. Other structures in the knee may also have been damaged, so make certain that you feel for areas of tenderness over the whole joint. Looseness or instability is sometimes difficult to evaluate. It must be confirmed by a physician, who should listen to your opinion.

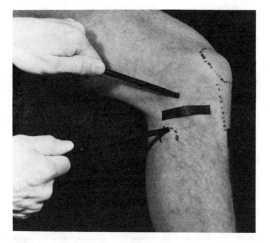

Figure 8-8. Location of outside (lateral) knee ligament tear.

Do's

- Use rest, ice, compression, and elevation **(Figures 8-9, 10, and 11)**.

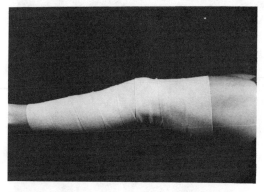

Figure 8-9.

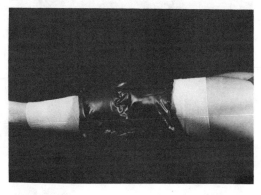

Figure 8-10.

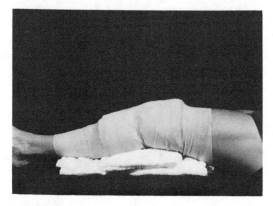

Figure 8-11.

- Splint and support the knee **(Figure 8-12)**.
- Bear weight if you are able without pain.

Don'ts

- Do not perform twisting or lateral movements of the knee, as they put stress on the injured ligament(s).
- Do not perform exercises in which the knee is rotated to a point at which the weight would pull on the ligament.
- *Do not* do exercise 1c if you have an outside (lateral collateral) ligament injury.
- *Do not* do exercise 1d if you have an inside (medial collateral) ligament injury.

Modifications

- Continue upper body weight training.
- Do exercises 1 through 6, to the point of pain (mild and moderate sprains *only*).

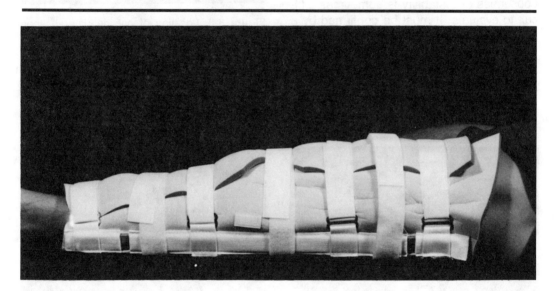

Figure 8-12. Immobilizing splint on knee.

Pain When Knee Extends

(Ligament Tears in Middle of Knee, Anterior Cruciate Ligament Tear)

The anterior cruciate ligament crosses in a diagonal pattern in the center of the knee, attaching the femur to tibia (**Figure 8-13**). Its purpose is to stop the lower leg from moving too far forward. Tearing of this ligament (**Figure 8-14**) is now considered to be one of the *most common knee injuries.*

A definite incident causes this problem. It usually results from a twisting motion when the foot of the injured leg is planted, with or without an extreme, quick straightening of the knee (hyperextension).

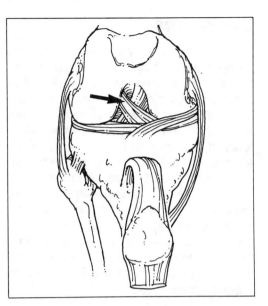

Figure 8-13. Anterior cruciate ligament crossing in knee.

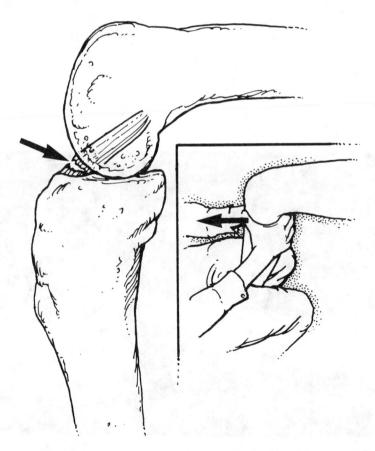

Figure 8-14. Torn anterior cruciate ligament allowing the tibia to move forward.

Symptoms

A loud "pop" may be heard when this injury occurs, and there may be a sensation that the knee is coming apart. The key symptom is rapid swelling of the knee. There is some pain when walking, and the knee feels "funny" or unstable. Other structures in the knee also may be involved (menisci or medial or lateral ligaments), so there may be specific areas of tenderness. If only the anterior cruciate ligament is torn, there will be no other areas of tenderness.

A "giving way" feeling of the knee will remain even after the injury has calmed down. The feeling will return whenever twisting and/or changing of direction movements are performed.

Do's

- Use rest, ice, compression, and elevation immediately after the injury occurs to avoid an extremely swollen and painful knee.
- Use a brace, or splint for support, as in **Figure 8-12**.
- Use crutches if walking is painful.

Don'ts

- Do not perform twisting or cutting movements.
- Do not fully straighten or hyperextend the knee **(Figures 8-15)**.

Modifications

- Continue upper body exercises.
- Continue straight line movements without pain.
- Do exercises 1 through 6, without pain. (Exercise 5 is the most important.)
- Remember: *DO NOT* completely straighten the knee during exercises, as this puts stress on the injured ligament.

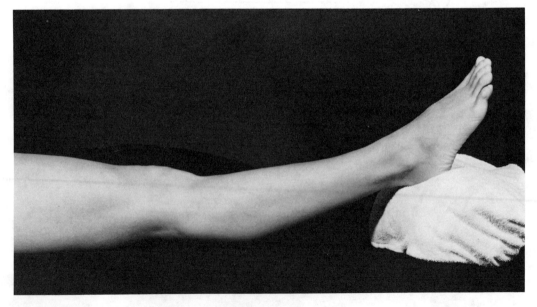

Figure 8-15. Fully straightened or hyperextended knee.

Ligament Tears in Back of Knee
(Posterior Cruciate Ligament Tear)

The posterior cruciate ligament crosses behind the anterior cruciate ligament in a diagonal pattern in the center of the back of the knee, attaching the femur to the tibia **(Figure 8-16)**. Its purpose is to stop the lower leg from moving backward **(Figure 8-17)**.

Tearing of the posterior cruciate ligament is very uncommon. It usually is caused by a direct blow to the front of the upper portion of the lower leg with the foot planted, rather than hyperextension of the knee, as experts previously thought. Hyperextension is more likely to produce an anterior cruciate ligament tear. Dashboard injuries resulting from a car accident frequently produce a posterior cruciate ligament injury.

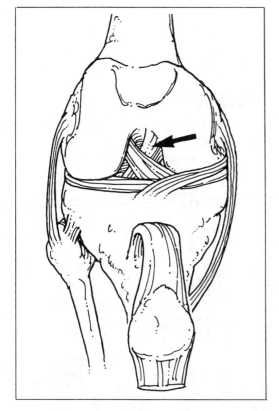

Figure 8-16. Posterior cruciate ligament crossing in knee.

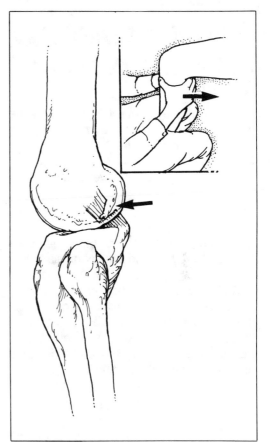

Figure 8-17. Torn posterior cruciate ligament, allowing lower leg (tibia) to move backward.

Symptoms

This is a difficult injury to identify. Swelling is not necessarily present. There is a feeling that something is not right in the knee, but it is hard to pinpoint the problem. There is no specific area of tenderness. A persistent feeling of looseness may tell you to seek medical advice.

Do's

- Use rest, ice, compression, and elevation.

- Continue upper body conditioning.
- Continue walking if you are free from pain.

Don'ts

- Do not perform twisting or cutting movements.

Modifications

- Do exercises 1 through 7, without pain.
- Double up on exercise 4; do less of 5.

Pain/Snapping on Side of Kneecap
(Plica)

A plica is a normal fold of soft tissue within the knee which may become thick and non-yielding **(Figure 8-18)**. Activity may irritate this band of tissue. A specific episode of injury does not have to occur.

Symptoms

When the knee bends, there may be a feeling of snapping in one particular location. If you put your hand on that spot, you may feel a snapping sensation. Sometimes, there is a sensation that the knee could lock. There is pain when you go up and down stairs, but there is little or no swelling. Frequently, there is just a general aching in the knee, especially after sitting for a period of time.

Do's

- Use rest, ice, compression, and elevation.

Don'ts

- Do not climb stairs excessively.
- Do not bend the knee repetitively.

Modifications

- Continue all activities to the point of pain.
- Do exercises 1, 3, and 7, without pain.

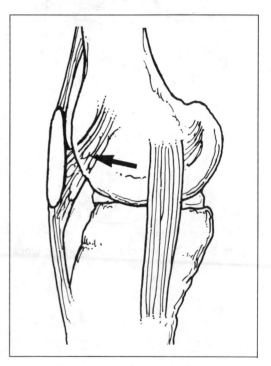

Figure 8-18. Knee plica (inner side view).

Torn Cartilage

The gristle-like substance (meniscus) that cushions the area where the femur sits on the tibia **(Figure 8-19)** can be torn. There are two cartilages in each knee (inside and outside), and tears can occur in either one, although the inside cartilage seems to be more vulnerable. Tears to the cartilage commonly occur when you cut or twist sharply or when you quickly and forcefully bend or straighten the knee. Meniscus tears rarely heal, because the blood supply to the cartilage is very poor. Surgical repair or removal may be necessary to restore normal, full movement.

Symptoms

There is tenderness along the "joint line" **(Figure 8-20)**. It is difficult to bend and straighten the knee. Often the knee may lock or catch, and it may feel like it is going to collapse. Swelling may sometimes be present in the back of the knee. Quick, cutting movements will be difficult. Also, you will be unable to fully squat (assume a deep knee bend position) without pain.

Do's

- Use rest, ice, compression, and elevation.

Don'ts

- Do not squat.
- Do not cause the knee to lock.

Modifications

- Continue all upper body conditioning.
- Do exercises 1 through 7, without pain.

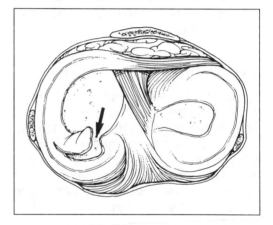

Figure 8-19. Torn cartilage (meniscus) in knee (view from the top).

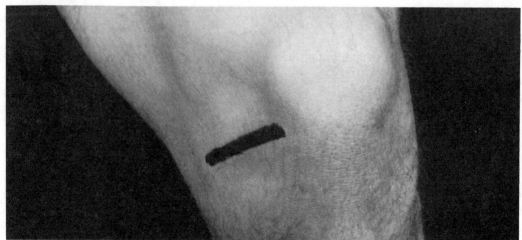

Figure 8-20. Location of tenderness, in area of joint line, when an inside (medial) cartilage is torn.

Pain Directly Behind Knee
(Baker's Cyst)

A cyst is a closed sac or pouch that contains fluid. Usually it is an abnormal structure. A Baker's Cyst is located behind the knee **(Figure 8-21)**, and it can usually be felt by pushing in on the area. Sometimes the cyst is large enough to see. It is a common problem in individuals of all ages. Baker's Cysts are almost always associated with other problems within the knee, such as torn cartilage or arthritis.

Symptoms

There may be pain and discomfort directly behind the knee. You may feel a small lump or see a small protrusion when the knee is completely straightened **(Figure 8-22)**. There may be some swelling behind the knee. Usually the condition is not caused by a direct incident or injury; rather, it results from problems inside the knee.

Do's

- Rest.
- Use ice, compression, and elevation.
- Continue all activity without pain.

Don'ts

- Do not do exercises that irritate this problem.
- Do not do squats.

Modifications

- Keep the legs strong to protect the knee.
- Do exercises 1 through 7, without pain.

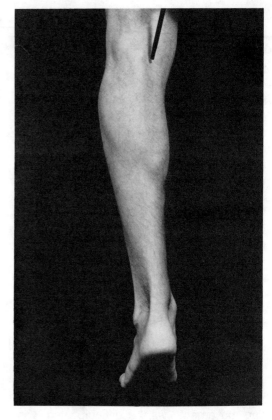

Figure 8-21. Location of Baker's Cyst, behind the knee.

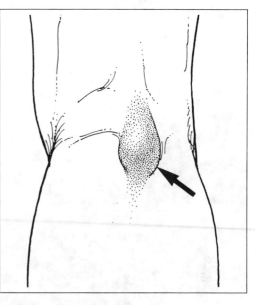

Figure 8-22. Visible protrusion behind knee (Baker's Cyst) when knee is fully extended.

Pain/Aching Inside the Knee
(Osteochondritis Dissecans)

Osteochondritis Dissecans is an unusual injury occurring in the middle of the knee. A piece of bone begins to separate, inside the knee, from the lower end of the thigh bone. Usually the condition begins gradually. The exact cause is sometimes unknown. One possible cause is a repeated injury to the knee. The piece of bone usually heals back in young individuals, otherwise the condition often requires surgery. If the piece separates completely, it may get caught in the joint, causing the knee to lock. The diagnosis can only be made after evaluating x-rays. Persons of any age can have this problem.

Symptoms

The knee will ache, and there may be general swelling. There may or may not be a specific incident or injury. The kneecap may catch or lock. Usually there is not a definite area of tenderness.

Do's

- Use rest, ice, compression, and elevation.
- Continue exercises, if they can be done without pain.

Don'ts

- If your knee locks, do not ignore this problem.

Modifications

- Emphasize strengthening the thigh muscles to prevent weakness and possible further injury to the knee.
- Do exercises 1 through 7, without pain.

Pain/Grating in Kneecap
(Chondromalacia)

Pain and grating in the kneecap (patella) area is usually a condition called chondromalacia, which is a gradual softening and/or roughening of the cartilage lining the undersurface of the kneecap **(Figure 8-23)**. This is not like a meniscus tear. Chondromalacia is a common knee problem that affects males and females of all ages who are physically active.

Symptoms

There is pain around the kneecap that is difficult to pinpoint. This may occur in one or both legs. A grinding sound and/or feeling is experienced when you bend the knee(s).

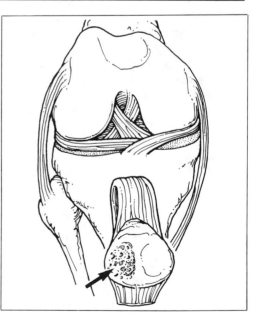

Figure 8-23. Chondromalacia of the kneecap (underside of the patella).

(Painless grinding is present in many normal knees and should not concern you.) Going up and down stairs and excessively bending and straightening your knees will cause pain. Tenderness is rare. Swelling around the kneecap does not occur at first, but may if the problem becomes chronic. This problem may get worse if exercises are not modified.

Do's

- Use rest, ice, compression, and elevation.
- Wear a knee support to hold kneecap in proper position **(Figure 8-24)**.

Don'ts

- Do not continue repetitive bending and straightening of the knee (with or without weights).
- Do not train using stair climbing.
- Do not do squat exercises—ever.

Modifications

- Continue all upper body weight training.
- Continue exercises 1, 3, 5, and 7 for the hamstrings.
- Do "end straightening" exercise 7 to avoid excessive bending and straightening of knee.

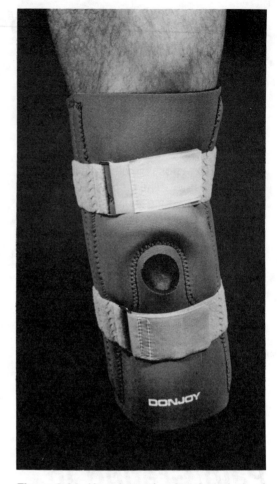

Figure 8-24. Knee brace for chondromalacia of the patella.

Dislocating or Subluxating Kneecap

The patella often moves partially or totally out of its normal position in front of the knee. Usually it moves to the outside (lateral side). If this problem is frequent and recurring, the undersurface of the kneecap will become irritated (see Chondromalacia).

Symptoms

The knee may feel like it is collapsing. You may fall down, or you may see the kneecap slip to the side of the knee, out of its normal position. Pain and swelling may be present, especially on the inside, slightly above the kneecap **(Figure 8-25)**. There may be a feeling of grating under the kneecap when you bend and straighten the knee.

Do's

- Use rest, ice, compression, and elevation.

Don'ts

- If kneecap is out of place, *do not* put it back—see a physician immediately.

Modifications

- Wear a kneecap brace, as in **Figure 8-24**.
- Do exercises 1 through 7, without pain. Emphasize exercise 4.

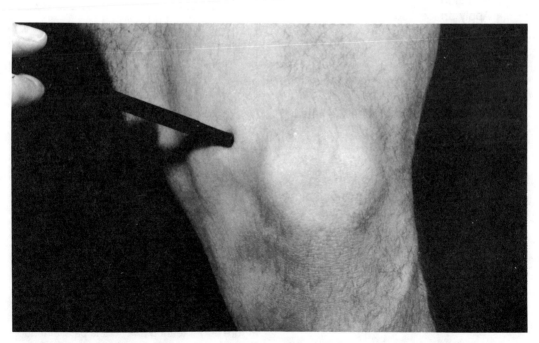

Figure 8-25. A common location of pain when kneecap moves out of its normal position.

Pain Below Kneecap
(Jumper's Knee, Patellar Tendinitis)

The patella attaches to the tibia by the patellar tendon **(Figure 8-26)**. Frequently overuse of the tendon through such exercises as jumping and heavy lower extremity weight training may cause some of this tendon to start tearing away from its attachment on the kneecap **(Figure 8-27)**.

Symptoms

There will be an area of pain and tenderness directly on the affected portion of the tendon. There will be pain after activity, and, if the problem progresses, during activity. There may be some minor swelling around the area of pain.

Do's

- Use rest, ice, compression, and elevation.
- Apply an ice cup.

Don'ts

- Do not ignore this problem—it will get worse.
- Do not continue activities like jumping if they are painful.

Modifications

- Avoid repetitive bending and straightening movements of the knee.
- Do exercises 1, 3, and 5 without pain.

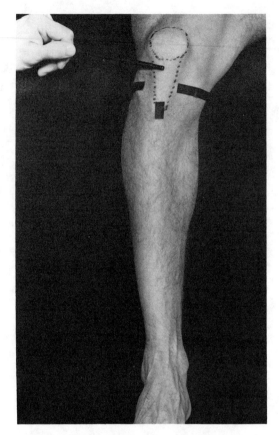

Figure 8-26. Location of patellar tendon.

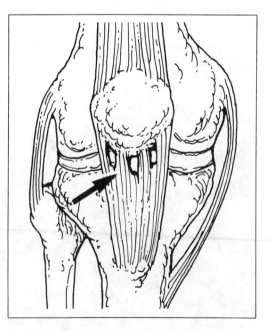

Figure 8-27. Tearing away of the patellar tendon from its attachment.

Pain Below Kneecap on Lower Leg Bone
(Osgood Schlatter's Disease)

The patellar tendon attaches the knee-cap to the tibial tuberosity **(Figure 8-28)** on the lower leg. In young athletes, this bony point on the lower leg is not completely hardened, because the skeleton's growth process is not finished. During activity, pulling of the patellar tendon on this weaker bony prominence may create soreness, tenderness, and swelling at the point of the tendon attachment **(Figure 8-29)**.

This problem occurs during the rapid growth years in adolescents and seems to occur more frequently in males. Once growth stops and the bone becomes hardened, the problem disappears, although a bump may remain where the tenderness occurred. This bump will be present for life. It is usually not painful unless it is injured.

Symptoms

There is specific pain directly over the area where the ligament attaches to the lower leg, and severe pain on kneeling, excessive jumping, or running. There may be local swelling and extreme tenderness.

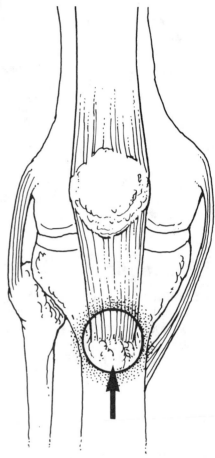

Figure 8-28. Attachment of the patellar tendon to the tibia at the tibial tuberosity.

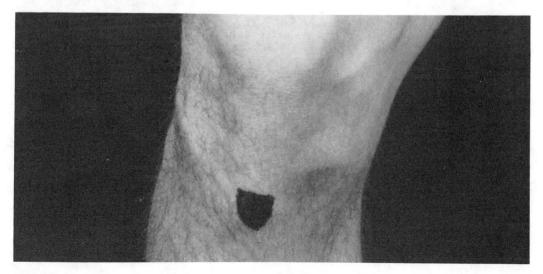

Figure 8-29. Location of pain in Osgood Schlatter's Disease.

Do's

- Use rest, ice, compression, and elevation.
- Apply an ice cup.
- Use a horseshoe-type pad to relieve tension on the tendon **(Figure 8-30)**.

Don'ts

- Do not kneel, as this produces severe pain.
- Limit extreme bending and straightening of the knee with weights or any type of resistance.
- Do not do squat exercises.

Modifications

- Continue all upper body weight training.
- Do not perform any activity that causes pain in this area.
- Do exercises 1, 3, and 5 without pain.

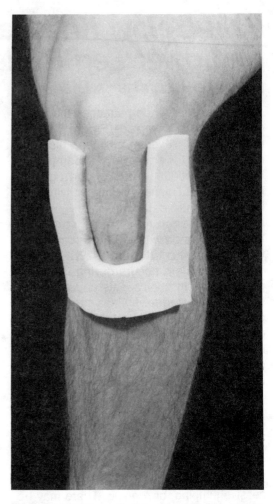

Figure 8-30. Horseshoe-type pad to relieve pressure at the point of irritation.

Pain/Snapping Over Outside of Knee
(Iliotibial Band Syndrome)

The iliotibial band is a thick, wide band of tissue running on the outside of the thigh, from the top of the hip, down across the knee, and attaching slightly below the knee on a bony prominence **(Figure 8-31)**. This band may become irritated through overuse, excessive running, or poor running mechanics. At times the band may move and snap back and forth during bending and straightening of the knee. This causes additional irritation where the band crosses the knee joint.

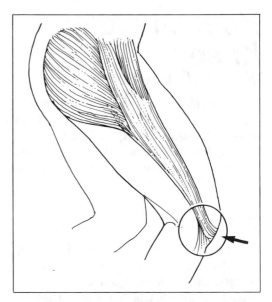

Figure 8-31. Location of the iliotibial band.

Symptoms

There is an area of tenderness on the side of the knee, where the band crosses the knee. Local swelling may be present, but it is unlikely. Pain and swelling increase if excessive bending and straightening of the knee continues.

Do's

- Use rest, ice, compression, and elevation.
- Apply an ice cup **(Figure 8-32)**.
- Use corrective inserts (orthodics) in shoes to improve running mechanics.

Don'ts

- Do not ignore this problem—it will get worse.
- Taping or bracing is not helpful.

Modifications

- Continue all upper body weight training.
- Limit excessive bending and straightening of the knee.
- Do exercises 1, 3, and 7, without pain.

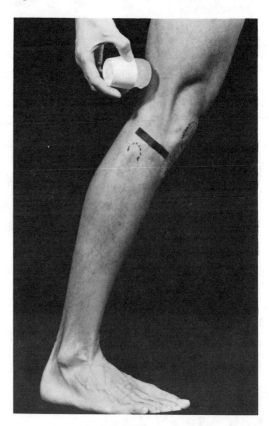

Figure 8-32. Applying an ice cup to the iliotibial band. Dark line marks joint line of knee, dotted line marks head of outside leg bone (fibula).

Housemaid's Knee
(Prepatellar Bursitis)

Prepatellar bursitis is an inflammation of the bursa that extends over the top of the kneecap **(Figure 8-33)**. It becomes inflamed after excessive kneeling activities. Usually, the problem goes away when the area is not under stress or pressure.

Symptoms

There is a definite area of pain directly over the affected area. There is specific swelling in the area of the pain, but not throughout the rest of the knee. There is also pain when pressure is applied to the swollen area.

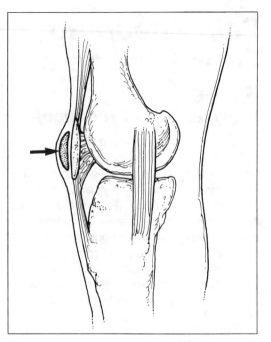

Figure 8-33. Location of prepatellar bursa.

Do's

- Use ice, compression, and elevation.
- Apply a donut-type pad to avoid pressure on the affected area.

Don'ts

- Avoid any kneeling activities.

Modifications

- Continue all upper body weight training.
- Continue all activities, if pain is not present.
- Do exercises 1, 3, 5, and 7, without pain.

Knee Exercises

The following exercises should be used with the problems discussed in this chapter. They are designed to restrengthen the musculature that surrounds the injured area to hasten recovery and ensure a safe return to activity. They will also help prevent injuries or injury recurrences. The exercises can be done anywhere, and no special equipment is needed. These exercises should be performed *without pain*, twice a day, as long as the problem is present.

Never do squats below a 90-degree angle of the knee **(Figure 8-34)**, as they will injure a healthy or problem knee. When doing this type of exercise, keep the back of the thigh (hamstrings) parallel to the ground **(Figure 8-35)**. *If possible, avoid squats altogether.*

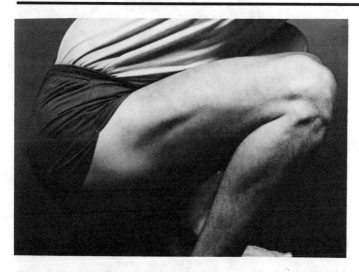

Figure 8-34. Incorrect "squats"—knees below a 90-degree angle.

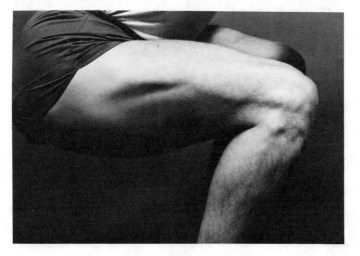

Figure 8-35. Correct "squats"—knees at 90-degree angle or hamstrings parallel to ground.

1. Straight Leg Raises

a. On your back, lean on your elbows. Lift one straight leg in a slow, controlled upward movement above the hip level **(Figure 8-36 and 37)**. Lower slowly. Do this 15 to 30 times, change legs, and repeat. Do this exercise twice daily.

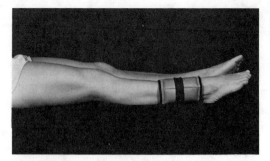

Figure 8-36.

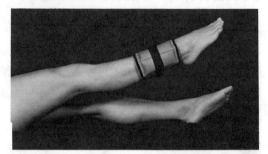

Figure 8-37.

b. Do the same exercise with leg moving out to the side **(Figure 8-38)**.

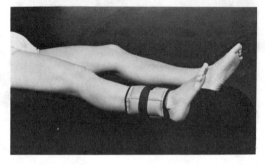

Figure 8-38.

c. Lie on your side, with both legs straight. Lift one straight leg in a slow, controlled upward movement **(Figure 8-39 and 40)**. Lower slowly. Do this 15 to 30 times, change legs, and repeat. Do this exercise twice daily.

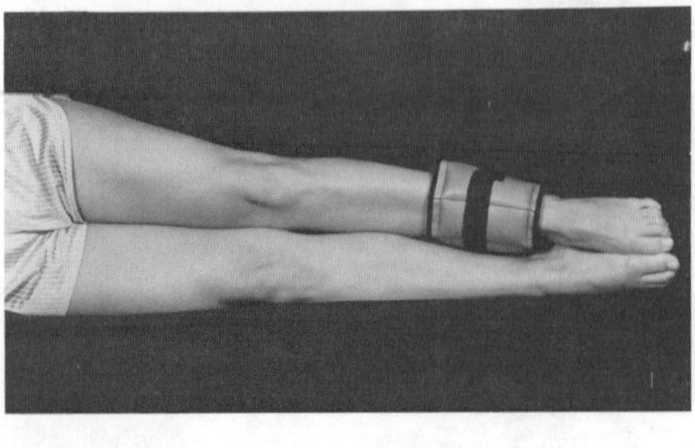

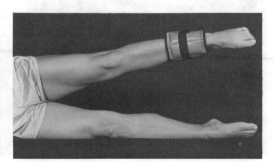

Figure 8-39.

Figure 8-40.

d. Lie on your side, with the top leg bent over your lower leg. Lift the bottom leg in a slow, controlled movement **(Figure 8-41 and 42)**. The inside of the lower ankle should be pointed at the ceiling. To make these exercises more difficult, add 1 to 5 pounds of weight to the lower leg while exercising. If you have an injury to the anterior cruciate ligament, keep both knees slightly bent during all exercises **(Figure 8-43 and 44)**.

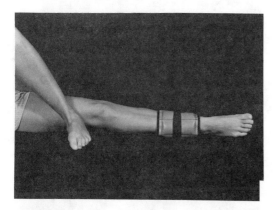

Figure 8-41.

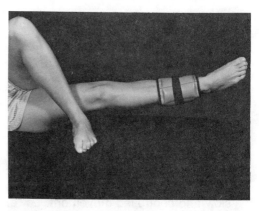

Figure 8-42.

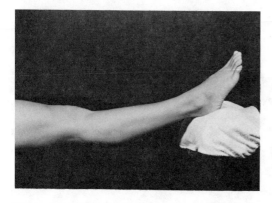

Figure 8-43. Wrong position—knee fully straightened.

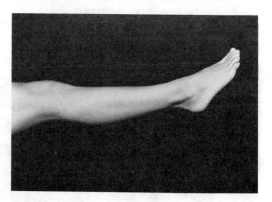

Figure 8-44. Correct position—knee slightly bent.

2. Hip Flexion Exercises

a. On your back, with one leg straight, bend other leg towards chest in a slow, controlled movement. Do this 15 to 30 times, then repeat with the opposite leg. Do this exercise twice daily **(Figure 8-45 and 46)**.

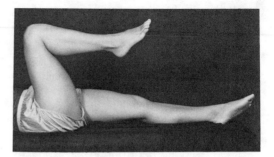

Figure 8-45.

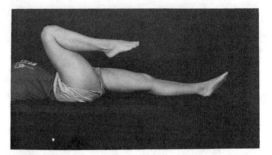

Figure 8-46.

b. Sitting in a chair with your feet on the floor, raise one knee to the chest in a slow and controlled movement. Lower slowly, change legs, and repeat **(Figure 8-47 and 48)**. Do this exercise 15 to 30 times, twice daily. To make exercises more difficult, add 1 to 5 pounds of weight to the leg being lifted.

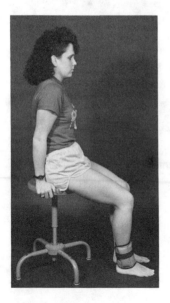

Figure 8-47.

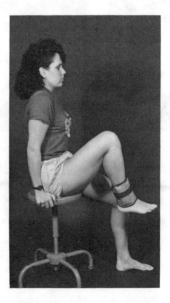

Figure 8-48.

3. Hip Extension Exercise

Lying on your stomach, with both legs straight, raise one straight leg in a slow, controlled movement above hip level **(Figure 8-49)**. Lower slowly. Do this 15 to 30 times, change legs, and repeat. Do this exercise twice daily.

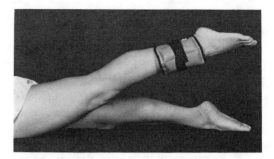

Figure 8-49.

4. Knee Extension

Sit with your legs over the edge of a table and your knees bent at right angles **(Figure 8-50)**. Lift one leg to a fully straightened position in a slow, controlled movement **(Figure 8-51)**. Lower slowly. Do 15 to 30 times, change legs, and repeat. Do this exercise twice daily. To make this exercise more difficult, add 1 to 5 pounds of weight to the leg being lifted. (If you have an injury to the anterior cruciate ligament, keep the knee slightly bent during all exercises, as shown in **Figure 8-43 and 44**).

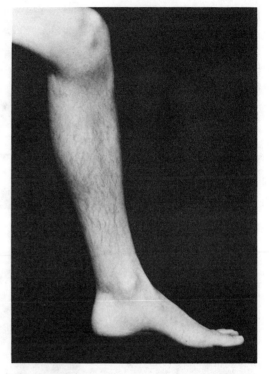

Figure 8-50.

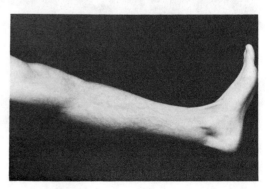

Figure 8-51.

5. Knee Flexion

Lie on your stomach, leaning on your elbows, with your legs straight **(Figure 8-52)**. Bend one leg to a right angle position in a slow, controlled movement **(Figure 8-53)**. Lower slowly. Do this exercise 15 to 30 times, change legs, and repeat. Do this exercise twice daily. To make this exercise more difficult, add 1 to 5 pounds of weight to the leg being lifted.

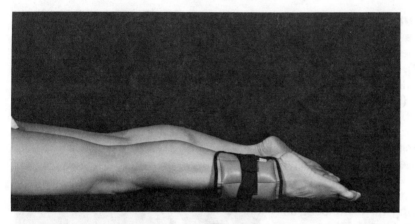

Figure 8-52.

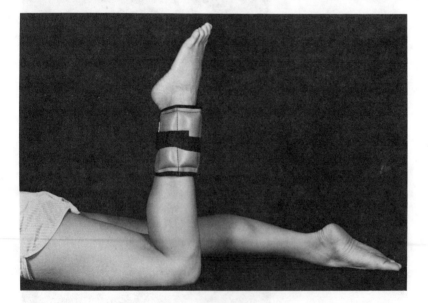

Figure 8-53.

6. Heel Raises

a. Stand with feet flat on the floor and arms down at your side. Raise heels and slowly go up on toes. Do this with feet in 3 positions:
1. Toes pointed straight ahead **(Figure 8-54)**. 2. Toes pointed in **(Figure 8-55)**. 3. Toes pointed out **(Figure 8-56)**. Repeat 10 to 20 times, twice daily.

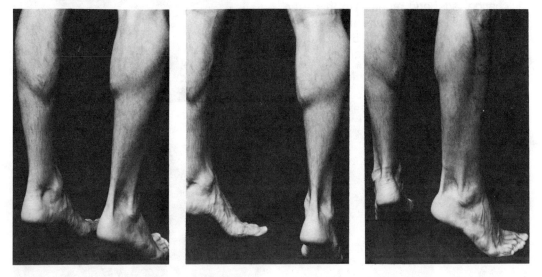

Figure 8-54.   Figure 8-55.   Figure 8-56.

b. Stand on a step, heels off the back edge, with hands on hips or out straight in front **(Figure 8-57)**. Drop heels below step **(Figure 8-58)**, slowly raise heels and go up on toes **(Figure 8-59)**, then slowly lower. Repeat 10 to 20 times, twice daily.

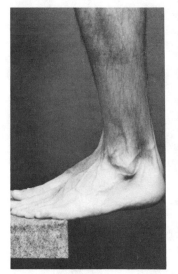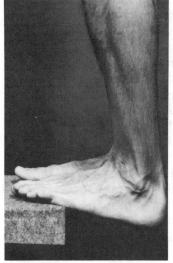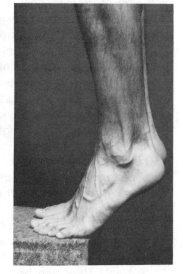

Figure 8-57.   Figure 8-58.   Figure 8-59.

7. End Straightening Exercises

Lie on your back with a towel roll under your knees **(Figure 8-60)**. Straighten one leg and move it upward in a slow, controlled movement **(Figure 8-61)**. Lower slowly. Do this 15 to 30 times, change legs, and repeat. Do this exercise twice daily. To make this exercise more difficult, add 1 to 5 pounds of weight to the leg being exercised.

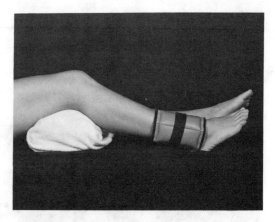

Figure 8-60.

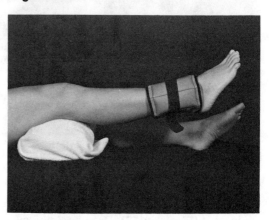

Figure 8-61.

8. Eccentric Loading Exercises

A type of exercise known as eccentric loading has proven to be extremely effective in the management of many chronic problems of the shoulder. This exercise series seems to relieve painful symptoms and hastens recovery time. Eccentric loading exercises emphasize a controlled range of motion, enabling the body part to be strengthened even when full range of motion is not present. They also stress muscle groups that do not perform the primary joint movement. The exercises restrengthen the area without risking re-injury or further overuse. These exercises (which are negative exercises) must be prescribed by a physician and taught by a physical therapist. They can be performed at home.

The Thigh

The thigh area **(Figure 9-1)** is surrounded by muscles that work both the hip and the knee. The muscles on the front of the thigh (quadriceps) cause the knee to straighten **(Figure 9-2)**. The muscles on the inside (medial) of the thigh (adductors) pull the entire leg toward the body **(Figure 9-3)**. The muscles on the back (posterior) of the thigh (hamstrings) bend the knee and straighten out the hip **(Figure 9-4)**. The muscles on the outside (lateral) of the thigh (abductors) pull the leg away from the body **(Figure 9-5)**.

The most common thigh problems are contusions in muscle tissue and tendon strains.

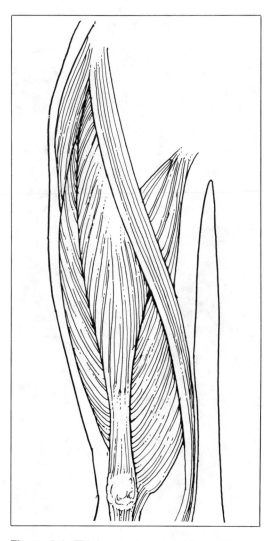

Figure 9-1. Thigh area between hip and knee.

Chapter **9**

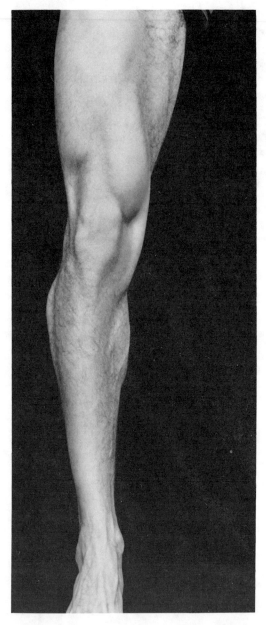

Figure 9-2. Muscles on front of thigh (quadriceps).

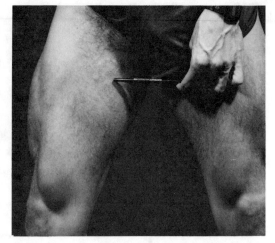

Figure 9-3. Muscles on the inside (medial-adductors) of the thigh.

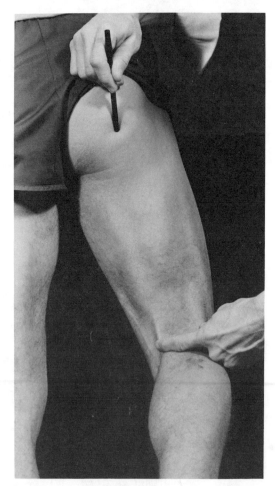

Figure 9-4. Muscles on the back (posterior-hamstrings) of the thigh.

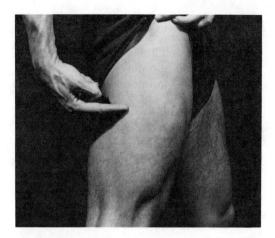

Figure 9-5. Muscles on the outside (lateral-abductors) of the thigh.

Discoloration In An Area
(Bruise, Contusion)

The most common location for thigh bruises is on the front of the thigh in the quadriceps. The quadriceps muscle starts in the area of the hip, goes down to join the kneecap, and continues to attach to the front of the lower leg. Bruises in this muscle are likely to occur in the large portion of the muscle, rather than at the tendons **(Figure 9-6)**.

Symptoms

There is a specific area of pain directly in the injured area. Usually discoloration is visible unless the bruise is very deep. There is a history of a direct contact or blow to the area. It might be difficult to bend and straighten the knee, since the muscle that performs those movements is injured.

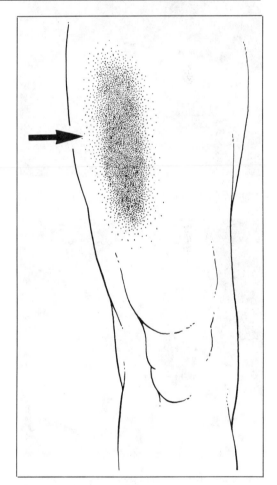

Figure 9-6. Most common location of thigh bruises—front of thigh (anterior-quadriceps).

Do's

- Use rest, ice, and compression **(Figure 9-7 and 8)** and keep the knee in a *bent position* when using ice and compression **(Figure 9-9)**. This keeps the muscle stretched so that it will not cramp. Bending also prevents blood from pooling around the injured area, which will help maintain a greater amount of normal motion at the knee as healing progresses.

Don'ts

- Do not keep the leg in a straight position while applying ice.
- Do not try to heavily exercise the injured leg.

Modifications

- Perform upper extremity weight training.
- Do the following mild thigh-stretching exercises without pain: 1a and b; 2a, b, and c; and 3a and b.

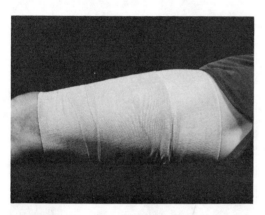

Figure 9-7. Compression wrap on bruised thigh.

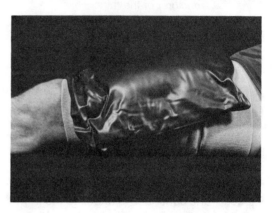

Figure 9-8. Ice pack on bruised thigh.

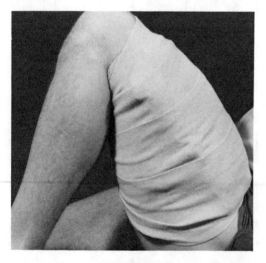

Figure 9-9. Knee in bent position when applying compression and ice. (Maintain this position when icing during the first few days following injury.)

Pain/Swelling in Muscle Area
(Myositis Ossificans, Bone Formation in Muscle)

After a deep bruise to a muscle has occurred, a pooling of blood may develop. This serious condition is called a hematoma. This area may turn to bone and limit knee motion for as much as a year **(Figure 9-10)**. You must try to prevent hematoma formation after a severe blow to the thigh by resting with the knee bent and using compression, ice, and elevation.

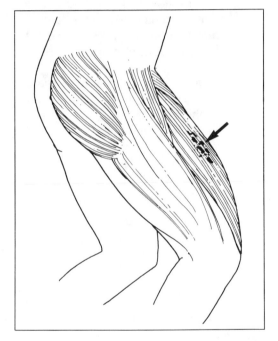

Figure 9-10. Pooling of blood in a bruised muscle that may turn to bone if treated improperly.

Symptoms

There will be an area of specific tenderness over the affected area. The discoloration may appear red rather than the usual black and blue. There will be some extreme swelling, tightness, and a feeling of hardness directly over the injured area. Stiffness and soreness may be present when you bend and straighten the knee.

Do's

- Use rest, ice, compression, and elevation with knee bent **(Figure 9-9)**. This must be done to avoid stiffness and pooling of blood.
- Wrap the thigh for support and compression.

Don'ts

- Stop all exercise (running, jumping, and lower extremity weight training).
- Do not massage the area—this may increase bleeding and pain.
- Always return to rest, ice, compression, and elevation with the knee bent, until swelling and pain have subsided.
- Do not resume activities until you have a complete range of motion.

Modifications

- Perform the following knee-bending and straightening exercises each day without pain: 1a and b; and 2a, b, and c.

Pain On Movement Of Muscle
(Strain, Muscle Tear)

Muscle strains can occur in any muscle of the body, but they most often occur in the quadriceps and the hamstring muscles of the thigh. There usually is a specific area of pain directly over the injured area. In mild tears, this pain might only be felt when the muscle is stretched or worked. In more severe tears, the pain may be constant. There may be stiffness when you bend and straighten the knee and/or when you move the leg in and out. Discolorations may appear in the injured area a few days after the injury. If a muscle tendon is completely torn, you will not be able to bend or straighten the knee normally.

Mild strains usually occur within the belly of the muscle, while more serious strains occur in the tendon. In the quadriceps, tears in the tendon often occur directly above the kneecap. In the hamstrings, tears often occur high, next to the buttocks, or low, just above the knee. In the inside of the thigh, tears occur close to the groin.

Muscle tears differ from general muscle soreness, which affects many muscle groups. A muscle tear occurs in a specific spot of a muscle. Muscle strains take time to heal—sometimes as much as 6 months to a year.

Do's

- Use rest, ice, compression, and elevation.
- Perform mild stretching without pain. This will keep the muscle stretched to prevent it from healing in a shortened position.

Don'ts

- Do not continue to use the muscle if symptoms linger—it needs rest.
- Do not overstretch.

Modifications

- Perform stretching exercises 1a and b for quadriceps strains; 2a, b, and c for hamstring strains; and 3a and b for abductor/adductor strains, without pain.
- Do exercises 4 through 8, without pain, to condition all major muscles of the thigh.

Thigh Exercises

The following exercises should be used with the problems described in this chapter. They are designed to restrengthen the musculature that surrounds the injured area to hasten recovery and ensure a safe return to activity. They will also help prevent injuries or injury recurrences. The exercises can be done anywhere, and no special equipment is needed. These exercises should be performed *without pain*, twice a day, as long as the problem is present.

1. Stretching Front of Thigh

a. Lie on your stomach, with your legs straight. Reach back and grasp the ankle of one leg. Gently pull it toward your buttocks **(Figure 9-11)**. Hold 5 to 8 seconds, repeat. Do this 5 to 10 times, change legs, and repeat. Do this twice daily.

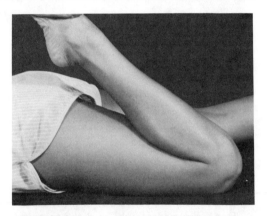

Figure 9-11.

b. Stand straight. Grasp one foot, bend your knee, and pull the foot towards your buttocks **(Figure 9-12)**. Hold 5 to 8 seconds, and repeat 5 to 10 times. Change legs and repeat. Do this twice daily.

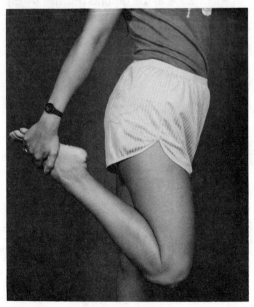

Figure 9-12.

2. Stretching Back of Thigh (Hamstrings)

a. Lie on your back, with your legs straight. Grasp one thigh, and gently pull it straight up **(Figure 9-13)**. Keep your hips flat and the other leg straight. Grasp the calf of your lifted leg, and pull it gently toward your chest **(Figure 9-14)**. Hold 5 to 8 seconds, and repeat 5 to 10 times. Change legs and repeat. Do twice daily.

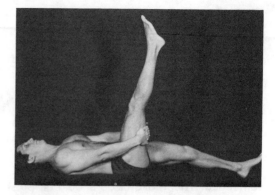

Figure 9-13.

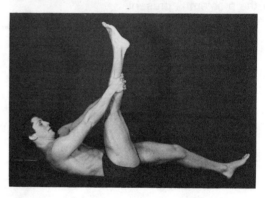

Figure 9-14.

b. Stand with your feet slightly apart. Bend forward slowly and try to touch your hands to the ground **(Figure 9- 15)**. Hold 5 to 8 seconds, and repeat 5 to 10 times, twice daily.

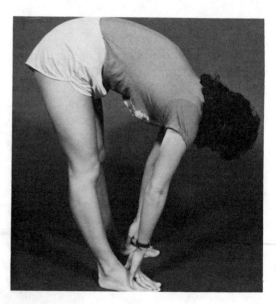

Figure 9-15.

c. Sit on the floor in a straddle position **(Figure 9-16)**. Lean forward over one leg, touching your chest to your knee **(Figure 9-17)**. Hold 5 to 8 seconds. Change sides and repeat. Do 5 to 8 times, twice daily.

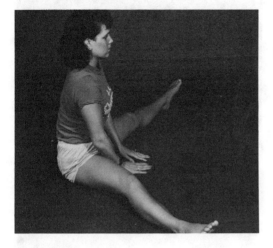

Figure 9-16.

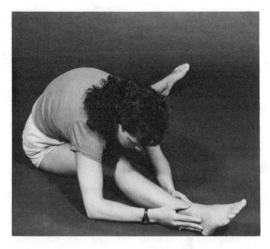

Figure 9-17.

3. Stretching Inside/Outside of Thigh (adductors/abductors)

a. Sitting on the floor, cross left leg over right. Lean forward, touching your head to the floor **(Figure 9-18)**. Hold 5 to 8 seconds. Repeat with right leg crossed over left. Do 5 to 10 times, twice daily.

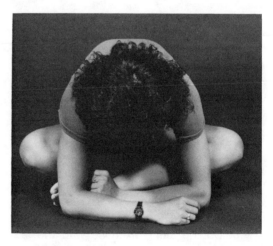

Figure 9-18.

b. Sit on the floor, with the soles of your feet together. Press your knees gently toward floor **(Figure 9-19)**. Hold 5 to 8 seconds. Do 5 to 10 times, twice daily.

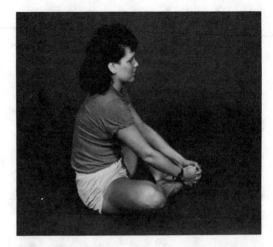

Figure 9-19.

4. Straight Leg Raises

a. On your back, lean on your elbows. Lift one straight leg in a slow, controlled upward movement above the hip level **(Figure 9-20 and 21)**. Do this 15 to 20 times, change legs, and repeat. Do this twice daily.

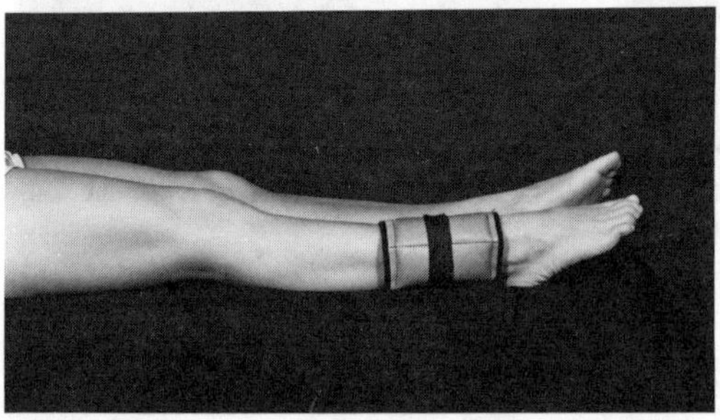

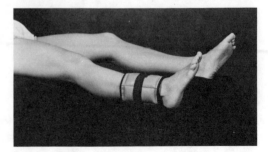

Figure 9-20.

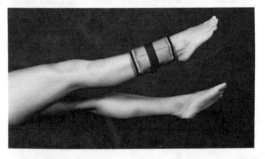

Figure 9-21.

b. Do the same exercise with the leg moving out to the side **(Figure 9-22)**.

Figure 9-22.

c. Lie on your side, with both legs straight **(Figure 9-23)**. Lift one straight leg in a slow, controlled movement **(Figure 9-24)**. Do this 15 to 20 times, change legs, and repeat. Do this twice daily.

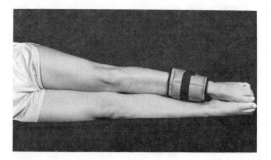

Figure 9-23.

Figure 9-24.

d. Lie on your side, with the top leg bent over the lower leg **(Figure 9-25)**. Lift the bottom leg in a slow, controlled upward movement. The inside of the ankle should be pointed up at the ceiling **(Figure 9-26)**. Do this 15 to 20 times, change legs, and repeat. Do this twice daily. To make these exercises more difficult, add 1 to 5 pounds of weight to the leg being lifted. (If you have an injury to the anterior cruciate ligament, keep the knee slightly bent during all exercises.)

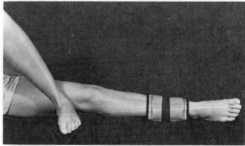

Figure 9-25.

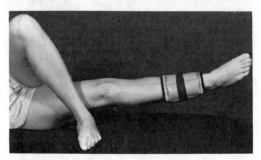

Figure 9-26.

5. *Hip Flexion Exercise*

a. Lie on your back, with one leg straight. Bend your other leg toward the chest in a slow, controlled movement **(Figure 9-27)**. Do this 15 to 30 times, and repeat with other leg. Do twice daily.

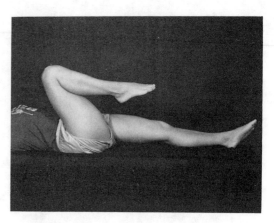

Figure 9-27.

b. Sitting in a chair, with feet on floor **(Figure 9-28)**, raise one knee to chest in a slow and controlled movement **(Figure 9-29)**. Change legs and repeat. Do this 15 to 30 times, twice daily. To make exercises more difficult, add 1 to 5 pounds of weight to the lower leg while exercising.

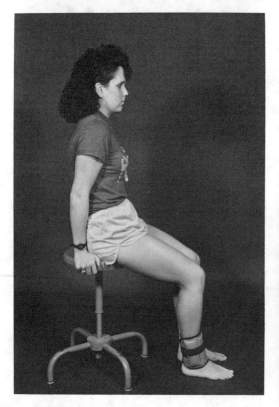

Figure 9-28.

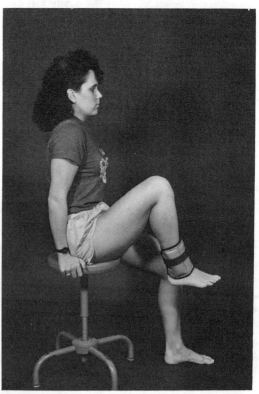

Figure 9-29.

6. *Hip Extension Exercise*

Lie on your stomach, with both legs straight **(Figure 9-30)**. Raise one straight leg in a slow, controlled movement, above hip level **(Figure 9-31)**. Do this 15 to 30 times, change legs, and repeat. Do this twice daily.

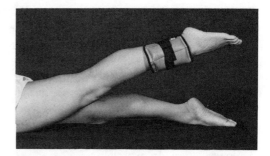

Figure 9-30.

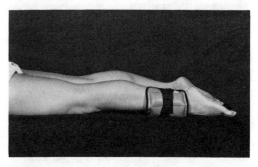

Figure 9-31.

7. *Knee Extension Exercise*

Sit with your legs over the edge of the table and your knees bent at right angles **(Figure 9-32)**. Lift one leg to a fully straightened position in a slow, con-trolled movement **(Figure 9-33)**. Do this 15 to 30 times, change legs, and repeat. Do this twice daily. To make this exercise more difficult, add 1 to 5 pounds of weight to the lower leg while exercising. (If you have an injury to the anterior cruciate ligament, keep the knee slightly bent during all exercises.)

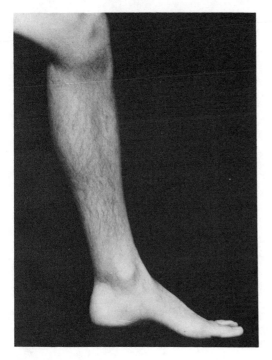

Figure 9-32.

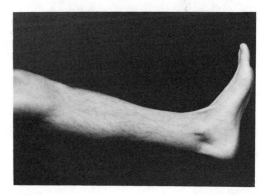

Figure 9-33.

8. *Knee Flexion Exercise*

Lying on your stomach, lean on your elbows, with your legs straight **(Figure 9-34)**. Bend one leg to a right angle position in a slow, controlled movement **(Figure 9-35)**. Do this 15 to 30 times, change legs, and repeat. Do this twice daily. To make this exercise more difficult, add 1 to 5 pounds of weight to the lower leg while exercising.

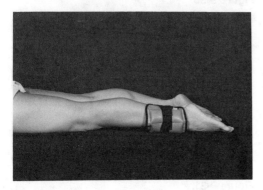

Figure 9-34.

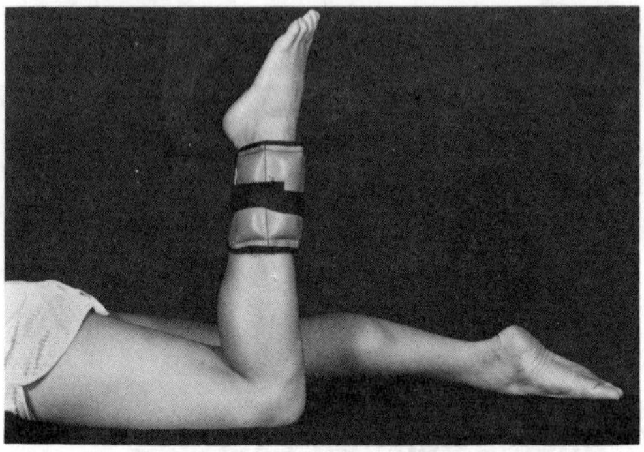

Figure 9-35.

The Hip

The hip is a joint which moves freely in many directions. It is strong, well-protected, and surrounded by several large muscles **(Figure 10-1)**. Problems at the hip joint are not very common, and they are usually easy to identify.

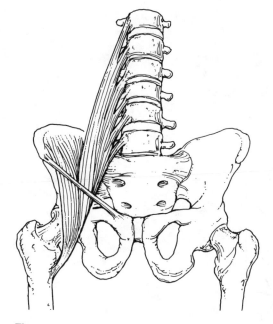

Figure 10-1. Hip joint surrounded by large muscle groups.

Chapter *10*

Pain in Front of Hip
(Iliopsoas Tendinitis, Avulsion Fracture, Stress Fracture)

Pain in the front of the hip (in the middle of the hip joint itself and possibly even in the groin area) may be caused by several conditions. The pain may be due to an inflammation of a tendon of a major muscle in the hip (iliopsoas tendinitis). It may be due to the same major tendon forcefully pulling off a small piece of bone at its attachment (avulsion fracture) **(Figure 10-2)**. It may even be due to a stress fracture (see Chapter 1).

All of these problems are caused by overuse—training too intensely, starting a training program too aggressively, or placing abnormal stresses on a particular area.

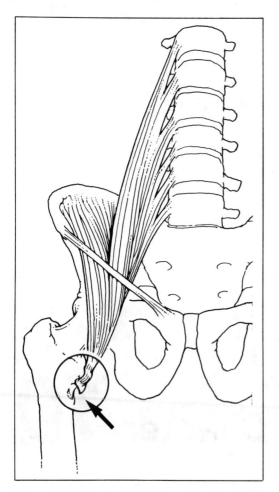

Figure 10-2. Tendon forcefully pulling off a small piece of bone at its attachment (avulsion fracture).

Symptoms

The symptoms of these problems are a deep, aching pain down in the middle of the hip joint. Pain will be present after and sometimes during activity. There is usually no swelling. It will be difficult to sit on the floor in a straddle position with your legs out to each side **(Figure 10-3)**. The problems will come on gradually. There will not be a specific injury incident. If symptoms persist, you may need an x-ray or even a bone scan to detect the problem.

Do's

- Rest.
- Use ice, compression, and elevation.
- Limit painful movements.
- Stop all activities if symptoms persist.

Don'ts

- Do not try to increase your activity when you have this type of pain.

Modifications

- Continue upper body exercises.
- Eliminate activities that cause pain.
- Do exercises 1a, b, and c; 2, and 3, without pain.

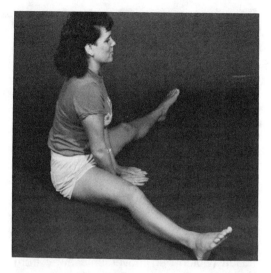

Figure 10-3. Sitting in straddle position may cause pain if a hip problem is present.

Pain on Outside of Hip
(Trochanteric Bursitis, Abductor Muscle Strain)

Pain on the outside of the hip can be due to an irritation of the bursa in that area. The problem occurs gradually. It is usually caused by too much pressure from excessive training, poor running form, or tight-fitting equipment. Occasionally this can be due to a direct blow.

The muscle that attaches to the bone can also be pulled or strained, producing a similar pain and a rather awkward gait. This injury is always associated with an abductor motion (violent leg movements away from the body).

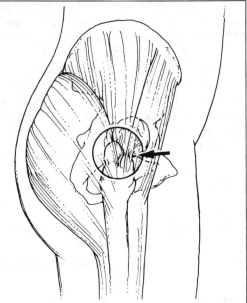

Figure 10-4. Pain on the outside of the hip due to irritation of the bursa.

Symptoms

The bony prominence on the outside of the hip **(Figure 10-4)** is painful. There may be pain when you move the hip in and out, or when you run on inclined surfaces. Usually there is no noticeable swelling.

Do's

- Rest.
- Apply ice bags. (It is difficult to apply compression and elevation to this area.)

Don'ts

- Do not increase your activity when you have this type of pain.
- Avoid tight clothing and pressure over the sensitive area.
- Avoid abductor exercises.

Modifications

- Continue upper body exercises.
- Eliminate activities that cause pain.
- Do mild stretching exercises: 1a, b, and c; 2; and 3, without pain.

Pain on Outside-Top of Hip
(Hip Pointer)

A hip pointer is a bruise to the outside portion of the pelvic girdle (illiac crest) **(Figure 10-5)**. It is caused by a direct blow to an area that is virtually unprotected. The muscles that attach to the pelvic girdle tighten and go into spasm. The injury also causes a severe pinching action to the soft tissues surrounding the area.

Symptoms

There will be severe pain directly over the injured area. It will be difficult to bend or twist the trunk since the muscles are tight and in spasm. There may be swelling and discoloration.

Do's

- Rest.
- Use ice and compression.

Don'ts

- Do not continue activities until the pain subsides. Hip pointers take weeks to heal.

Modifications

- Pad this area for protection when you return to activity.

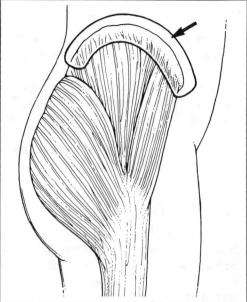

Figure 10-5. Location of bruise to the top of the hip (hip pointer).

Snapping on Side of Hip
(Snapping Tensor Fascia Lata)

This problem may occur when you bend or rotate the hip joint. It usually takes place when a large band of fascia or tendon moves over the side of the hip bone (greater trochanter) with a snapping sensation **(Figure 10-6)**. The onset of symptoms is gradual, but if the problem is ignored, the area will become very irritated. This injury is common in ballet dancers.

Symptoms

The hip feels like it pops out of place. You can actually see something jump over the outside of the hip. If the activity continues, there is increasing pain and soreness in the affected area.

Do's

- Rest.
- Use ice and compression.

Don'ts

- Do not do activities that cause pain.

Modifications

- Do hip stretching exercises 1a, b, and c; 2; and 3, without pain, to keep the muscles from tightening.

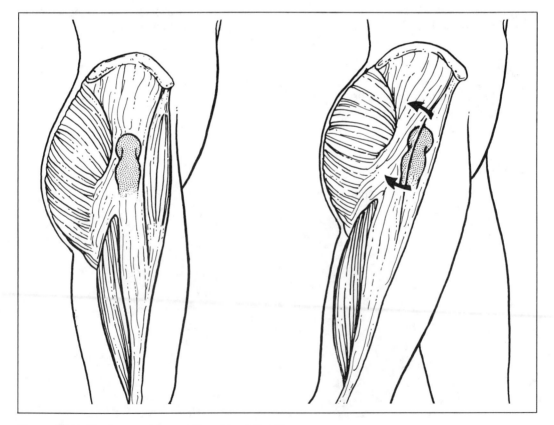

Figure 10-6. Tendon moving over the side of the hip.

Buttocks Bruise

A bruise to the buttocks is caused by a direct blow or contact. Blood vessels are ruptured, and bleeding occurs underneath the skin, causing discoloration.

Symptoms

There is a specific area of pain directly over the injured area **(Figure 10-7)**. Discoloration is frequently present. There may be some stiffness during movement. There is history of direct contact or a blow to the area.

Do's

- Rest.
- Apply ice.

Don'ts

- Do not continue activities that are painful.

Modifications

- Do hip-stretching exercises 1a, b, and c.

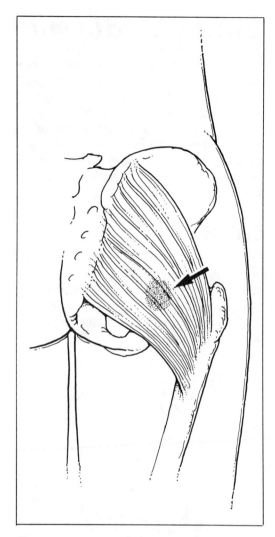

Figure 10-7. Bruise to buttocks.

Buttocks Bursitis

Pain in the lower portion of the buttocks may be caused by an irritation of the bursa located around the bone on which you sit (ischial tuberosity) **(Figure 10-8)**. It may be irritated by a direct fall on the bottom or by activities that cause pressure in this area. Lower buttock pain without a known injury could be coming from a back problem. In this situation, consult a physician.

Symptoms

There is specific pain on the area where the bursa is located. Sitting is uncomfortable, and it may be painful to bend and straighten the knee because the muscle behind the hamstring muscles attaches to the bony prominence.

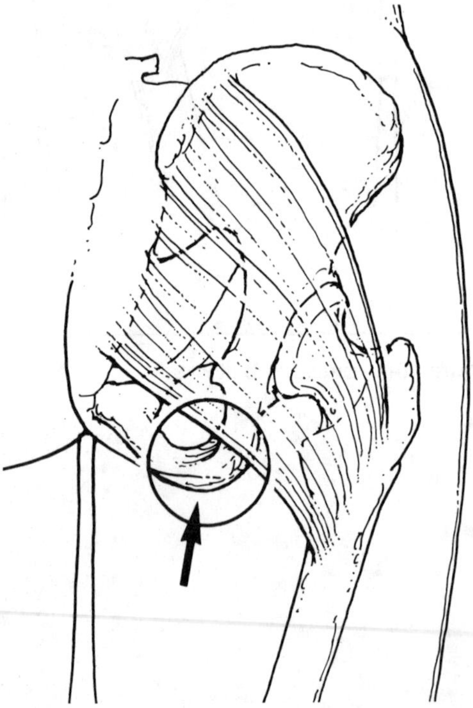

Do's

- Rest.
- Apply ice.
- Use a pad or donut when sitting.

Don'ts

- Do not do activities that cause pain.
- Avoid any extreme contact to area.

Modifications

- Do hip-stretching exercises 1a, b, and c; 2; and 3; without pain.

Figure 10-8. Location of pain in lower portion of buttocks due to irritation of the bursa located in that area.

Hip Exercises

The following exercises should be used with the problems described in this chapter. They are designed to restrengthen the musculature that surrounds the injured area to hasten recovery and ensure a safe return to activity. They will also help prevent injuries or injury recurrences. Following injury, they should be started as soon as they can be performed correctly, without pain. Pain should never be present during these exercises. The exercises can be done any-where, and no special equipment is needed. These exercises should be performed 2 to 3 times a day, as long as the problem is present.

---

1. Hip Stretching Exercises

a. Stand straight. Grasp one foot, bend your knee, and pull the foot towards the buttock of the same leg **(Figure 10-9)**. Hold 5 to 8 seconds, and repeat 5 to 10 times. Change legs and repeat. Do this twice daily.

b. Sitting on the floor, cross left leg over right. Lean forward, touching your head to the floor. Hold 5 to 8 seconds **(Figure 10-10)**. Repeat with right leg crossed over left leg. Hold 5 to 8 seconds. Do 5 to 10 times, do twice daily.

c. Sit on the floor, with the soles of your feet together. Gently press knees to floor **(Figure 10-11)**. Hold 5 to 8 seconds. Do 5 to 10 times, twice daily.

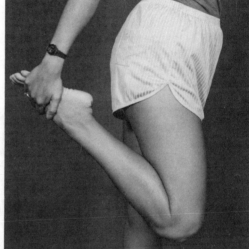

Figure 10-9.

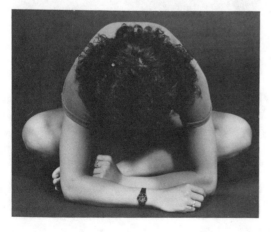

Figure 10-10.

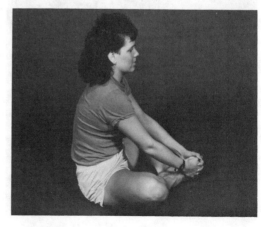

Figure 10-11.

2. Hip Flexion Exercises

a. Lie on your back, with one leg straight. Bend your other leg toward the chest in a slow, controlled movement **(Figure 10-12 and 13)**. Do this 15 to 30 times, and repeat with the other leg. Do twice daily.

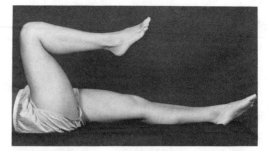

Figure 10-12.

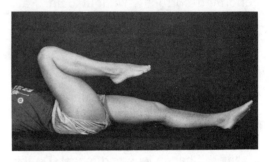

b. Sitting in chair, with feet on floor **(Figure 10-14)**, raise one knee to chest in a slow and controlled movement **(Figure 10-15)**. Change legs and repeat. Do this 15 to 30 times, twice daily. To make exercises more difficult, add 1 to 5 pounds of weight to the lower leg while exercising.

Figure 10-13.

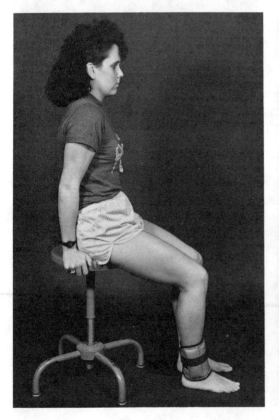

Figure 10-14.

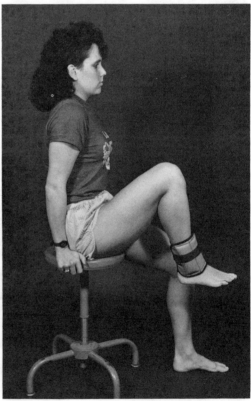

Figure 10-15.

3. Hip Extension Exercise

Lie on your stomach, with both legs straight **(Figure 10-16)**. Raise one straight leg in a slow, controlled movement, above hip level **(Figure 10-17)**. Do this 15 to 30 times, change legs, and repeat. Do twice daily.

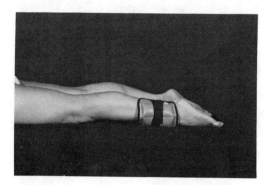

Figure 10-16.

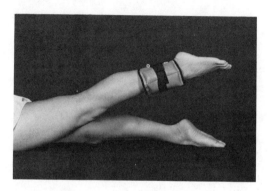

Figure 10-17.

The Abdomen

The abdomen (stomach area) contains many muscles that protect the internal organs. These muscles proceed from the back, the side, and the chest **(Figure 11-1)**. Like any other muscle, they may be bruised or strained.

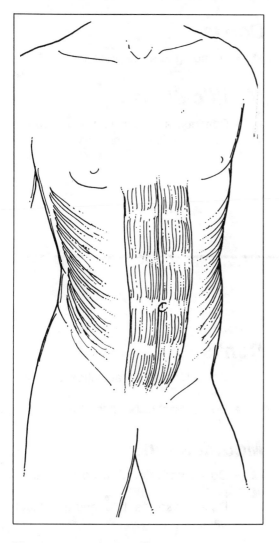

Figure 11-1. Abdomen area.

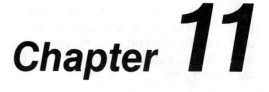

Chapter **11**

Pain/ Discoloration in Stomach Area
(Bruises to the Abdomen)

While abdominal bruises are generally treated like bruises in any other muscle group, you must be alert for injury to the internal organs. These muscles protect such organs as the liver, kidneys, spleen, and intestines. Bruises to these internal organs can be serious and even life-threatening. Any significant bruise to the abdomen is potentially dangerous; it should be watched very closely.

Symptoms

There is a specific area of pain in the abdominal area where contact was made. A specific incident caused the injury. Some tightening of the muscles in the area (muscle spasm) may occur, and it may be difficult to bend or rotate the trunk. If any internal organs are injured there will be continued pain in the stomach area, nausea and/or vomiting, and possibly blood in the stool or urine.

Do's

- Rest.
- Apply an ice pack to the affected area.
- If symptoms indicate possible injury to internal organs, see a physician immediately.

Don'ts

- Do not ignore the problem.

Modifications

- Continue all activities if you have no pain or serious symptoms.

Muscle Strains in Abdomen

Abdominal muscle strains are usually caused by sudden twisting or reaching movements. The muscles may begin cramping and cause spasms in the area. In a muscle strain, there is a *specific* area of pain, unlike general muscle soreness, which produces stiffness throughout the entire muscle area.

Do's

- Rest.
- Use ice and compression.

Don'ts

- Do not continue activities that are painful.
- Do not twist or bend the trunk.

Modifications

- Do all activities that do not cause pain.
- Do exercises 1a, b, c, and d, without pain.

Pain in Side
(Stitch in Side)

A "stitch in the side" is a cramp-like pain which develops on the left or right side of the abdominal area during exercise **(Figure 11-2)**. This can be a very uncomfortable problem which may cause you to stop activity momentarily. The exact cause of the muscle spasm is not known. It sometimes is attributed to food eaten before exercise or to weak abdominal muscles.

Do's

- Do not eat heavily before activity.
- When the problem occurs, stretch the arm on the affected side as high as possible, or bend the upper body forward. Applying direct pressure on the affected area with your hand may also help.
- Strengthen your abdominal muscles.

Don'ts

- Do not ignore this problem if it recurs—see your physician.

Modifications

- Do exercises 1a, b, c, and d without pain.

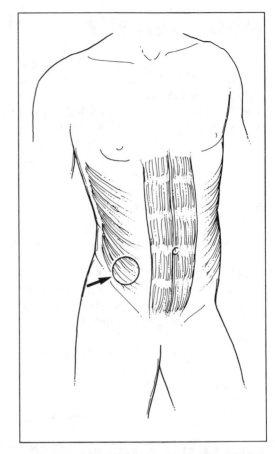

Figure 11-2. Location of cramp-like pain in the side of the abdomen that develops during exercise (stitch in the side).

Abdominal Exercises

The following exercises are ones which should be used with the previous problems. They are designed to restrengthen the musculature that surrounds the injured area to hasten recovery and ensure a safe return to activity. They will also help prevent injuries or injury recurrences. Following injury, they should be started as soon as they can be performed correctly, without pain. Pain should never be present during these exercises. The exercises can be done any-where, and no special equipment is needed. These exercises should be performed 2 to 3 times a day, as long as the problem is present.

1. Abdominal Curl

a. Lie on your back with your knees bent and feet flat. Put your hands behind your head, elbows out straight. Raise your shoulders off the floor, less than halfway toward your knees **(Figure 11-3)**. Do not bend up to your knees; stop less than halfway. Lower slowly and relax. Do this 15 to 20 times, twice daily.

b. Do the same exercise as above, with your arms crossed across your chest **(Figure 11-4)**.

c. Do the same exercise as above, with your hands behind your head, pointing (but not touching) your elbow to the opposite knee, alternately **(Figure 11-5)**.

d. Do the same exercise as above, with knees bent toward chest at a 90-degree angle **(Figure 11-6)**.

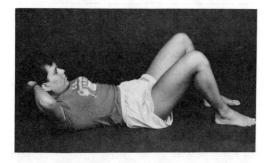

Figure 11-3.

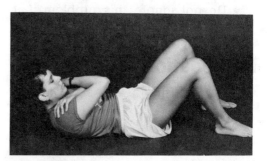

Figure 11-4.

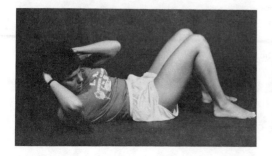

Figure 11-5.

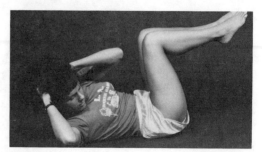

Figure 11-6.

The Thorax

The thorax is usually known as the chest. The ribs serve to protect the vital organs found in the chest and to help the lungs during breathing **(Figure 12-1)**.

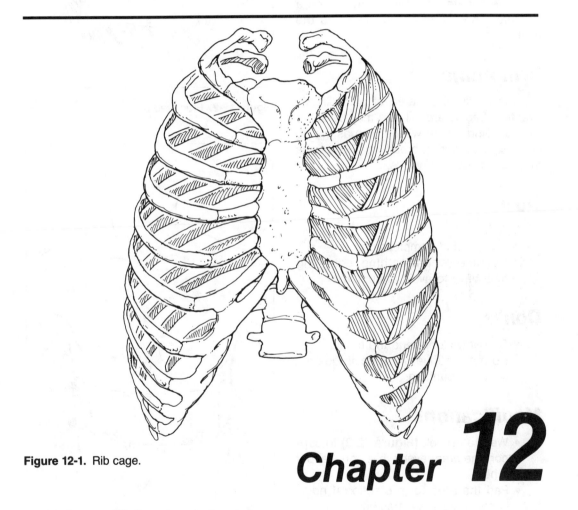

Figure 12-1. Rib cage.

Chapter 12

Pain in Ribs
(Rib Bruises and Fractures)

The ribs are flat bones which attach to the upper back bone in the back and to the breast bone (sternum) in the front. Ribs can be bruised or fractured **(Figure 12-2)**. The causes and symptoms of these problems are similar. In most cases, there has been a direct blow. Some rib injuries may result from violent contractions of the muscles that attach to the ribs. (The contractions can be caused by forceful coughing.) Only an x-ray can differentiate between a bruise and a fracture. The treatment, however, is the same.

Symptoms

There will be an area of pain directly over the affected area. There may be some local swelling. There will be pain as the rib cage expands during breathing. Symptoms may last for several weeks.

Do's

- Rest.
- Use ice and compression.
- Practice deep breathing, coughing frequently to avoid pneumonia.

Don'ts

- Do not twist or bend the trunk.
- Do not continue painful activities except for coughing.

Modifications

- Wear a rib belt **(Figure 12-3)** to support the area, even while you sleep if it helps.
- Pad the area for protection if additional contact is expected.

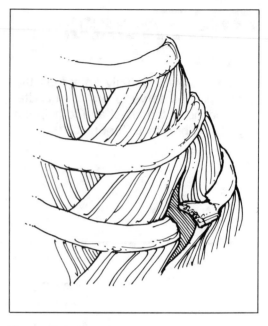

Figure 12-2. Fractured rib.

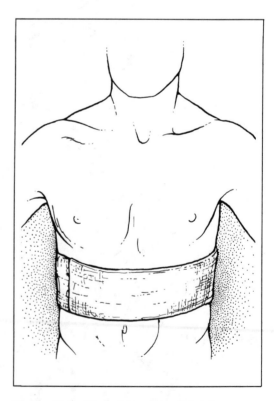

Figure 12-3. Rib belt to support rib injury.

Injury to Internal Organs

The same forces that produce injury to the ribs can also cause injury to the internal organs that the rib cage protects. These may include the kidneys, liver, spleen, or bladder. Injury to these organs can be extremely serious resulting in a life-threatening medical emergency.

Symptoms

There is a history of a significant blow or force delivered to the thorax area and/or abdomen. Pain will be present in the area of the blow or directly over the affected internal organ. Symptoms which indicate serious injury may include nausea or vomiting, signs of shock, or blood in the urine. These symptoms may occur within a short time following the injury or may appear a day or two following injury.

Do's

- Apply ice to affected area in 30-minute intervals over 48 to 72 hours following injury.
- Contact a physician or go to a hospital immediately if any of the previously mentioned symptoms are present.

Don'ts

- Do not continue physical activity if internal injury is suspected.
- Do not continue any weight training.

Modifications

- Pad the affected area when returning to activity, if further contact is expected.

Other injuries related to thorax injuries are discussed in chapters dealing with the shoulder and abdomen.

The Low Back

The low back includes the vertebrae (bony segments of the spinal column) from below the rib cage to the tail bone **(Figure 13-1)**. The low back area is the site of frequent problems. These problems can become very complicated, making physician consultation necessary.

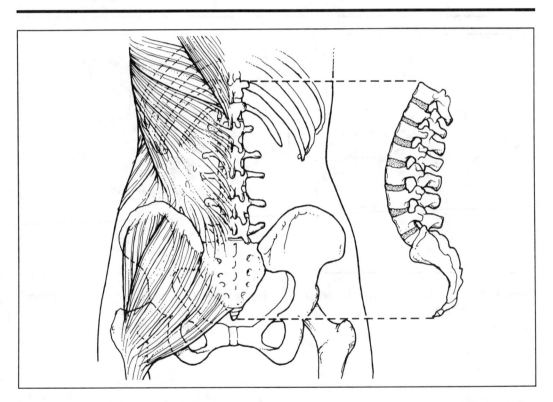

Figure 13-1. Low back area, including bony segments (vertebrae) from below the rib cage to the tail bone.

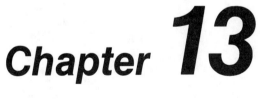

Chapter *13*

Pain in the Low Back
(Disc Problems: Intervertebral Disc Syndrome, Ruptured Disc, Herniated Disc)

In the area between two vertebral bones is a rigid cartilage substance containing a disc (jelly-like center) **(Figure 13-2)**. Its purpose is to absorb shock. When the disc material protrudes out of its normal area, it may put pressure on the surrounding nerves and cause pain **(Figure 13-3)**. Protrusions may be caused by a variety of factors. Disc problems generally take several weeks to resolve and may require surgery.

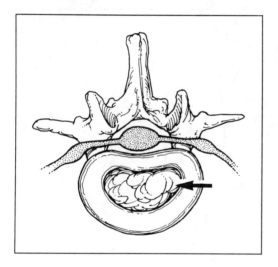

Figure 13-2. Disc in back located between each vertebra.

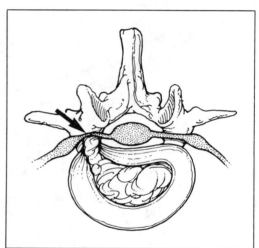

Figure 13-3. Disc protruding out of its normal area, putting pressure on the surrounding nerves.

Symptoms

There is pain in the low back **(Figure 13-4)**, in the area of the affected disc, and tightness in the surrounding muscles. There may be pain radiating into the buttock, down the back of the leg, and sometimes into the heel or to the front of the foot. Pain may be worse during coughing, sneezing, or straining on the toilet. Any movement of the low back is painful. There may be a feeling of muscle weakness in the area. Lying on your back with your knees bent may be more comfortable. Strengthening the stomach muscles will help to support the low back area.

Do's

- Rest.
- Apply ice on the painful area.

Don'ts

- Do not continue activities, as you may stimulate more muscle spasms.

Modifications

- Use low back support when sitting or driving.
- Rest on your flattened back with your knees bent.
- Do exercises 1a, b, and c; 2; 3; 4; and 5, without pain.

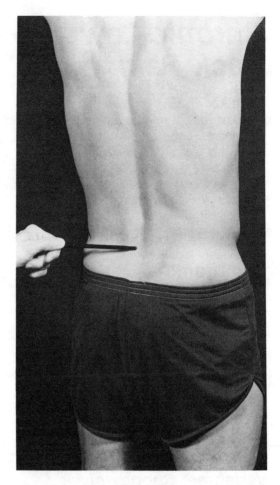

Figure 13-4. Common location of pain in low back area.

Chronic Low Back Pain

The origin of most chronic low back pain is unknown, but muscle strains, abnormal movements, and poor posture may contribute to this problem. The low back muscles may become tight and painful. Such movements as twisting and lifting will cause low back pain to worsen or recur. Strengthening the stomach and back muscles will help to support and protect the low back area.

Symptoms

In the area of the low back there will be pain. The muscles surrounding the low back will be tight. There may be pain in the buttocks, but it will not radiate down the leg. Motion is restricted.

Do's

- Rest.
- Do not continue activities, as you may stimulate muscle spasms.
- Do not twist or jerk your back.

Modifications

- Use low back supports when sitting and driving.
- Rest on your flattened back with your knees bent.
- Do exercises 1 through 5, without pain.

Sharp Pain in Low Back
(Stress Fracture of Vertebrae, Spondylolysis, Spondylolisthesis)

Repeated stress to a particular area in the low back may cause a stress fracture (spondylolysis) in a portion of the vertebra **(Figure 13-5)**. If it is not treated, the weakened vertebra begins to slip forward and separate from its normal position (spondylolisthesis) **(Figure 13-6)**. These problems are usually provoked by movements that hyperextend the back. Gymnastic activities, weight lifting, tennis, and the butterfly swim stroke are common sources of these overuse problems. The onset of symptoms is gradual and usually begins in early adolescence.

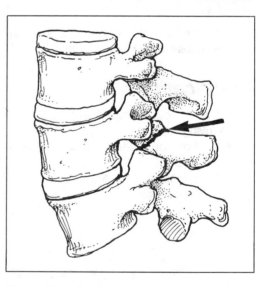

Figure 13-5. Fracture in a portion of a vertebra (spondylolysis).

Symptoms

There may be general low back pain on one or both sides of the back, along with some muscle tightness. Backward bending exercises may be painful. A direct blow or sudden twist may cause the vertebra to slip, creating a specific area of pain directly over the affected vertebra with occasional pain radiating into the buttocks and legs. Bending forward, even to a mild degree, is impossible.

Do's

- Rest.
- Apply ice.
- Decrease your activity level.
- Consult a physician if pain persists.

Don'ts

- Do not ignore the problem.
- Do not continue activities that are painful.

Modifications

- Do back exercises 1 through 5 without pain.

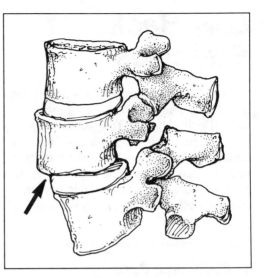

Figure 13-6. Slippage and separation of vertebra from its normal position (spondylolisthesis).

Fractured Vertebra

Fractures can occur in any vertebra. A fracture to this area can be caused by a direct blow or contact, or by a forceful muscle contraction.

Symptoms

There will be pain directly on the affected area as well as muscle tightness on both sides of the back. Bending and straightening the back will cause intense pain. Pain may radiate into the buttocks and the back of the legs.

Do's

- Rest.
- Apply ice.
- Consult a physician if pain persists.

Don'ts

- Do not continue activities that are painful.

Modifications

- Do not perform any special exercises until the area has healed.

Low Back Exercises

The following exercises are ones which should be used with the problems discussed in this chapter. They are designed to restrengthen the musculature that surrounds the injured area to hasten recovery and ensure a safe return to activity. They will also help prevent injuries or injury recurrences. Following injury, they should be started as soon as they can be performed correctly, without pain. Pain should never be present during these exercises. The exercises can be done anywhere, and no special equipment is needed. These exercises should be performed 2 to 3 times a day, as long as the problem is present.

1. Abdominal Curls

a. Lie on your back with your knees bent and feet flat. Put your hands behind your head, elbows out straight. Raise your shoulders off the floor, less than halfway toward your knees **(Figure 13-7)**. Lower slowly and relax. Do this 15 to 20 times, twice daily.

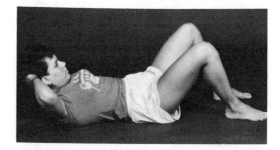

Figure 13-7.

b. Do the same exercise as above, with your arms crossed across your chest **(Figure 13-8)**.

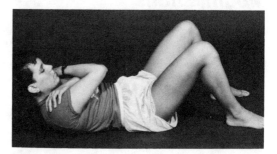

Figure 13-8.

c. Do the same exercise as above, with your hands behind your head, pointing (but not touching) your elbow to the opposite knee, alternating **(Figure 13-9)**.

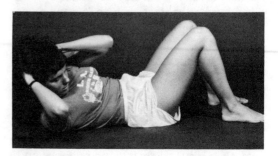

Figure 13-9.

2. Pelvic Tilt

Lie on your back, with your knees bent and your feet flat on the floor **(Figure 13-10)**. Roll your hips and pelvis back toward you and push lower back flat to floor **(Figure 13-11)**, hold for 5 seconds, and relax. Repeat 10 to 15 times, twice daily.

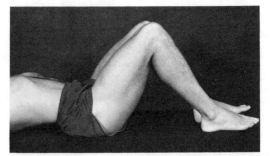

Figure 13-10.

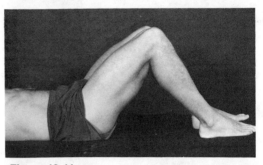

Figure 13-11.

3. Alternate Knee to Chest

Lie on your back with your legs straight and together. Grasp one knee and pull it gently to your chest, keeping your other leg straight **(Figure 13-12)**. Hold this position for 5 seconds, and relax. Change legs and repeat. Do this 10 to 15 times, twice daily.

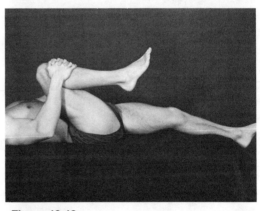

Figure 13-12.

4. Press-Up Exercise

Lie on your stomach with your hands by your shoulders in a push-up position. Slowly raise the chest, keeping your hips on the floor **(Figure 13-13)**. Hold this position 5 seconds, and relax. Do this 10 to 15 times, twice daily.

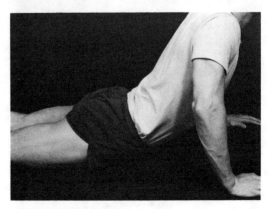

Figure 13-13.

5. *Hamstring Exercises*

Lie on your back with your legs straight. Grasp one thigh, and pull it gently toward your chest, keeping your hips flat and the other leg straight **(Figure 13-14)**. Grasp the calf of the lifted leg, and pull it gently toward your chest **(Figure 13-15)**. Hold this position for 5 seconds, and relax. Change legs and repeat. Do this 10 to 15 times, twice daily.

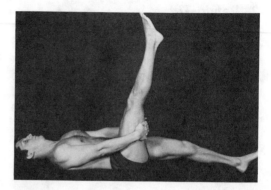

Figure 13-14.

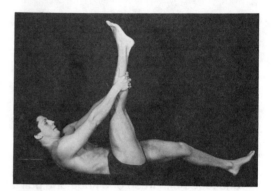

Figure 13-15.

The Neck

The neck consists of muscles, ligaments, and vertebra **(Figure 14-1)** between the shoulders and the head which protect the spinal cord **(Figure 14-2)**. When problems occur, pain can be felt in the neck, shoulder, arm, or hand.

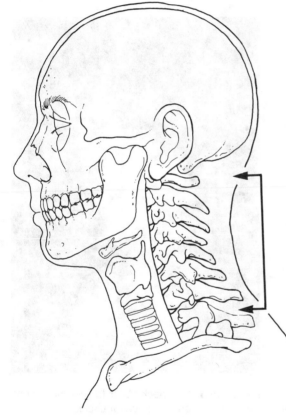

Figure 14-1. Vertebrae of the neck.

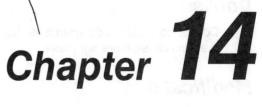

Chapter **14**

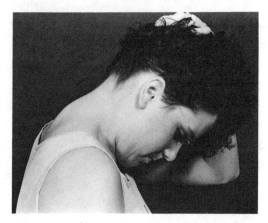

Figure 14-2. Neck area.

Stiffneck
(Wryneck, Torticollis)

This common problem happens without direct injury to the neck. You may wake up with this problem after sleeping on the neck the wrong way. Exposure to a draft or holding the head in an unusual position for a long time may also produce a stiffneck.

Symptoms

There is stiffness and muscle tightness on one side of the neck. Head movement is limited.

Do's

- Apply heat.
- Mildly massage the neck.
- Perform neck-stretching exercises.

Don'ts

- Do not do upper body exercises, as they will cause more tightness.

Modifications

- Wear a soft neck collar to limit movement and help relax muscles **(Figure 14-3)**.

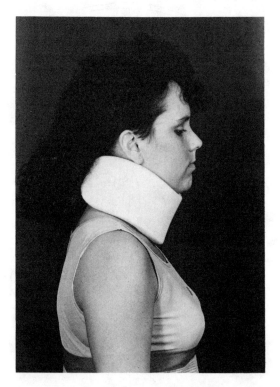

Figure 14-3. Soft neck collar to limit movement and rest neck muscles.

Burning Pain Down Neck/Arm
("Burner", Pinched Nerve, Cervical Nerve Stretch Syndrome)

This is a potentially serious problem in which a nerve in the neck is stretched or pinched. It can occur if you receive a blow to the side of the head or neck that violently twists the neck to the side **(Figure 14-4)**.

Symptoms

A burning, knife-like pain radiates from the neck, down the arm, and possibly into the hand. There may be some numbness and loss of movement in the arm and hand. These symptoms usually last only seconds, leaving the arm weak and sore for a variable time afterwards.

Do's

- Rest.
- Apply ice.
- Wear a support collar.

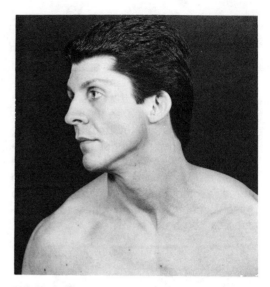

Figure 14-4.

Don'ts

- Do not continue activities until this condition is evaluated by a physician.

Modifications

- Perform exercises 1 and 2 to strengthen the neck, only after there are no symptoms.

Neck Sprain
(Whiplash)

A neck sprain occurs from a violent forward or backward snapping of the head and neck. The supporting muscles and ligaments are injured.

Symptoms

There is usually pain in the neck at the time of the injury, but pain can get worse the next day. Head and neck movement is limited and uncomfortable. The muscles in the area are tight and in spasm. This problem may take weeks and even months to heal.

Do's

- Rest.
- Apply ice.

Don'ts

- Do not continue activities if they are painful.

Modifications

- Wear a soft collar to support and protect neck.
- Do exercises 1 and 2, without pain.

Neck Exercises

The following exercises should be used with the previous problems. They are designed to restrengthen the musculature that surrounds the injured area to hasten recovery and ensure a safe return to activity. They will also help prevent injuries or injury recurrences. Following injury, they should be started as soon as they can be performed correctly, without pain. Pain should never be present during these exercises. The exercises can be done anywhere, and no special equipment is needed. These exercises should be performed 2 to 3 times a day, as long as the problem is present.

1. Neck Stretching

Sit or stand with your arms straight down. Move your neck in a slow, controlled pattern forward, backward, left, and right. Your ears should touch your shoulders in the latter movements. Do this 10 to 15 times, twice daily.

2. Neck Strengthening

Sit or stand. Using your hand(s) as resistance, move your head in all directions, pushing it in the opposite direction of the force of your hand(s) **(Figure 14-5 to 7)**. Do this exercise 10 times each direction, twice daily.

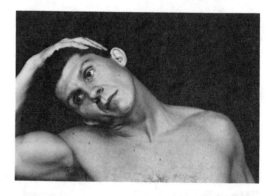

Figure 14-5.

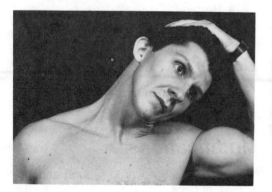

Figure 14-6.

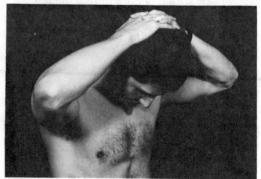

Figure 14-7.

The Shoulder

The shoulder is a joint that moves in nearly every direction. The bones of the shoulder are held together by ligaments, and the entire shoulder complex is supported by several large muscle groups **(Figure 15-1)**.

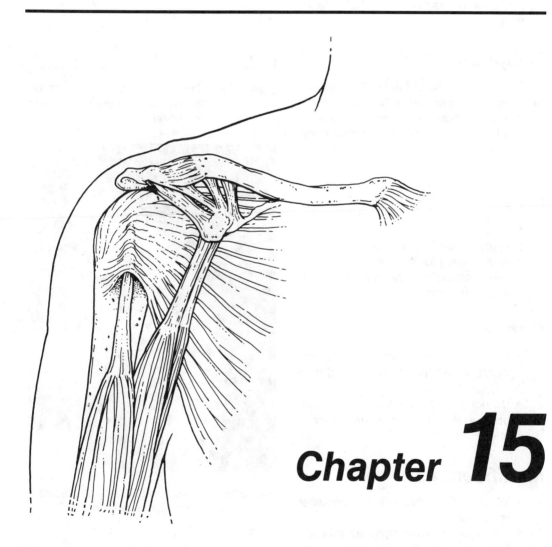

Chapter 15

Figure 15-1. Shoulder complex showing bones, ligaments, and muscles.

Pain on Top of Shoulder
(Shoulder Separation, Acromioclavicular Separation, AC Separation)

Injuries to the top of the shoulder usually involve ligaments connecting the collarbone (clavicle) to the top of the shoulder **(Figure 15-2)**. Falling on the shoulder or on an outstretched arm can stretch or tear these ligaments, allowing the clavicle to ride high, sometimes coming completely out of the joint.

Symptoms

There is an area of tenderness directly over the prominent bone **(Figure 15-3)**. There is pain when you move the shoulder, and it may even hurt to let the arm hang straight down, as this pulls on the injured ligament.

Do's

- Rest.
- Apply ice and compression.
- Wear a sling for support.
- See a physician. This condition may require surgery.

Don'ts

- Do not try to move the shoulder too much, unless this is encouraged by a physician.
- Do not do activities that cause pain, unless this is encouraged by a physician.

Modifications

- Wear a sling whenever the shoulder is painful.
- Continue lower extremity exercises.
- Do exercises 1, 2, 3a and b, 4, 5a and b, 6, 7, and 8, without pain.

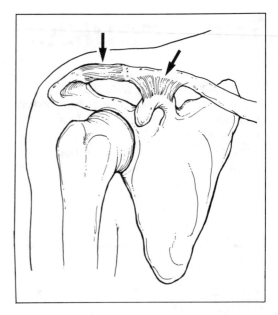

Figure 15-2. Ligaments on the top of the shoulder commonly injured in a shoulder separation.

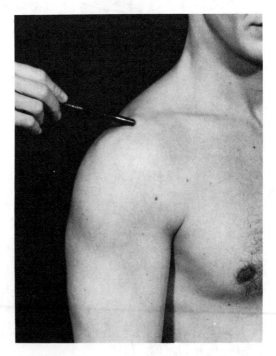

Figure 15-3. Location of pain may be present in a shoulder separation.

Pain in Muscles Of Shoulder
(Rotator Cuff Tear)

The rotator cuff is a group of 4 large muscles which surround the shoulder **(Figure 15-4)**. These muscles can tear if there has been a violent pull to the arm, a forceful twisting, or a fall on an outstretched arm. Strains may also be caused by repetitive stress in the shoulder through throwing or heavy weight lifting.

Symptoms

Shoulder movements are painful, and some may be difficult or impossible to do. The pain may be directly over the injured muscle or tendon area. This problem may last for several months.

Do's

- Rest.
- Apply ice and compression.
- Perform easy range of motion exercises if they are tolerable.

Don'ts

- Do not continue activities that are painful.

Modifications

- Use a sling if it relieves pain.
- Continue lower extremity exercises.
- Do exercises 1, 2, 3a and b, 4, and 5a and b, without pain.

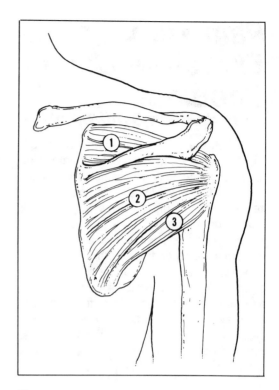

Figure 15-4. Three of the 4 rotator cuff muscles which surround the scapula.

Pain with Excessive Use of Shoulder
(Impingement Syndrome)

When the shoulder is overused, swelling may occur in the area of the rotator cuff, decreasing the space in which the rotator cuff muscles move. When this space is limited and the shoulder moves, a portion of those muscles becomes irritated, especially when the arm is lifted out to the side in a horizontal plane and above the head. Such movements are common in the butterfly swim stroke and in many throwing, hitting, and lifting techniques. Since the impingement syndrome is difficult to control, you can expect it to last for several months. Sometimes surgery is necessary to enlarge the space.

Symptoms

There is aching and pain in the shoulder as the arm moves above shoulder level. Sometimes the aching is worse at night. Pain is not present at any specific point. It can be difficult to move the arm across the body and to touch the opposite ear or shoulder. It may be painful to bring the arm back into a throwing position. While warm-ups will decrease the pain, continuous use will bring it back. Discomfort worsens after activities stop.

Do's

- Rest.
- Apply ice.

Don'ts

- Do not continue activities that are painful, or this problem will get worse.

Modifications

- Perform shoulder exercises 1 through 5 without pain.
- Limit arm movement so that activities are not painful.
- Change techniques to avoid stress in the shoulder.

Shoulder Out of Place
(Dislocation, Subluxation)

In the shoulder, dislocations occur where the upper arm (humerus) meets the rest of the shoulder complex **(Figure 15-5)**. When a subluxation or dislocation occurs, ligaments, tendons, and muscle tissue are torn. Usually, the injury is caused by a direct blow or a fall on an outstretched arm.

Unfortunately, dislocations are likely to recur. Therefore, the initial treatment should be aggressive. See a physician for an x-ray and, possibly, a procedure known as a reduction, which moves the bone back into place. You could break a bone or injure a nerve by attempting a reduction yourself.

After a 1st reduction, do not move the shoulder for 3 to 6 weeks. Immobilization is not as important after a 2nd dislocation and reduction. You may need to have the shoulder surgically repaired.

Symptoms

There is severe pain in the affected shoulder and tightness (spasm) in the surrounding muscles. A visible deformity is noticeable, because the injured shoulder does not look like the non-injured one. You are unable to touch the opposite shoulder with the hand of the affected arm, and you prefer immobility. If the shoulder is only subluxated, movement is possible but painful.

Do's

- Immobilize the shoulder with a sling if possible.
- Apply ice.
- See a physician immediately—the shoulder must be put back in place as soon as possible.

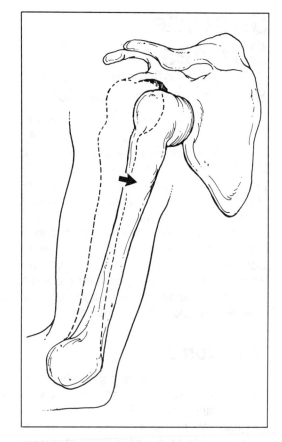

Figure 15-5. Shoulder dislocation—upper arm (humerus) moves totally out of its normal position.

Don'ts

- Do not let anyone, other than a physician, try to put the shoulder back in place.

Modifications

- Perform exercises 1 through 8 without pain.

Shoulder Stiffness
(Shoulder Inflammation, Bursitis, Frozen Shoulder)

Bursitis of the shoulder is an inflammation of the bursa in the area **(Figure 15-6)**. The problem develops gradually. A specific injury or overuse may cause shoulder stiffness. Sometimes bursitis stems from another problem in the shoulder, such as a ligament or muscle tear.

There may be so much inflammation in the joint that it becomes stiff and "frozen." Soft tissues in the shoulder become damaged. If you properly care for problems in the shoulder when they begin, you will most likely avoid a frozen shoulder.

Symptoms

Shoulder movements, especially movements away from the body or throwing motions, are painful. Motion may become progressively restricted. There is an aching sensation when you rest or do not move the shoulder. Symptoms appear gradually. The muscles may feel weak.

Do's

- Rest.
- Apply ice.
- Do active motion.

Don'ts

- Do not continue activities that are painful unless directed by a physician or therapist.

Modifications

- Perform exercises 1 through 5 without pain.
- Infrequently, a physical therapist needs to help get the shoulder moving.

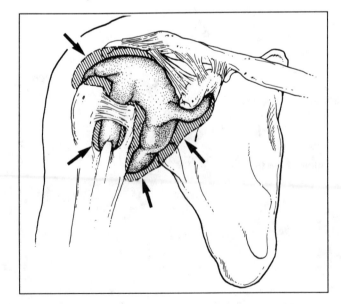

Figure 15-6. Inflamed bursa in shoulder (bursitis).

Pitcher's Shoulder
(Osteochondritis Dissecans, Overuse)

Excessive use of the shoulder in a young adolescent (in throwing or pitching activities, for example) can eventually damage the surfaces of the shoulder joint. Sometimes small fragments of bone break loose and move about inside the joint. If these pieces become lodged in a certain position, they may cause the joint to lock. This problem occurs gradually.

Symptoms

There is pain in the shoulder when you throw. You may notice an aching sensation after activity. The shoulder may "lock" on occasion.

Do's

- Rest.
- Apply ice.

Don'ts

- Do not continue excessive activity.

Modifications

- Continue lower extremity activities.
- Complete thorough warm-ups before activities.
- Change your throwing pattern to avoid pain.
- Do exercises 1 through 8 without pain.
- If symptoms do not improve, see a physician.

Pain/Aching Down Arm
(Thoracic Outlet Syndrome)

Thoracic Outlet Syndrome occurs when the nerves, arteries, and veins are compressed as they come from the spine and chest to the arm. Muscle spasm in the area is one cause of this problem. Symptoms are produced by abnormal pressure on 1 or all 3 of the structures. The syndrome may last for several days and tends to recur.

Symptoms

There is pain and aching down the arm, into the hand. You may notice impaired circulation, a cold sensation in the hand, and tingling in one or more of the fingers. Muscles of the arm or hand may be weak. The problem is not necessarily associated with any particular movement, but it is often related to a certain position that the shoulder and neck are in.

Do's

- Rest.
- Apply ice.
- Use a sling support to relieve tension.
- Move your neck to correct an abnormal position.

Don'ts

- Do not continue activities that are painful.

Modifications

- Maintain proper posture. For example, do not let your shoulders droop.
- Do exercises 1 through 3 without pain.

Pain on Collarbone Attachment to Breast Bone
(SC Sprain [Sternoclavicular Sprain])

There are ligaments that connect the clavicle to the sternum. Injury to these ligaments is called a SC Sprain **(Figure 15-7)**. This potentially serious problem may be due to a direct blow or extreme twisting movement with the arm going backward.

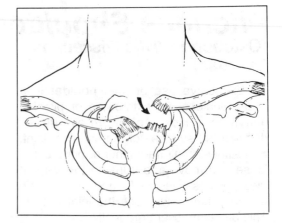

Figure 15-7. Tear (sprain) of the ligament connecting the clavicle to the sternum (SC sprain).

Symptoms

There will be pain directly over the injured joint **(Figure 15-8)**. Swelling may be present. The end of the clavicle may look deformed. You will not be able to move your arm across your chest or pull your shoulders back without pain. If the clavicle moves in towards the neck, there will be hoarseness.

Do's

- Rest.
- Apply ice.
- See a physician. This condition could be dangerous and may require surgery.

Don'ts

- Do not continue exercises that are painful.
- Do not continue upper body exercises.

Modifications

- Perform exercises 1 through 5 without pain.

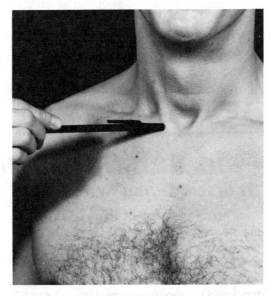

Figure 15-8. Location of pain when SC sprain occurs.

Shoulder Exercises

The following exercises should be used with the problems discussed in this chapter. They are designed to restrengthen the musculature that surrounds the injured area to hasten recovery and ensure a safe return to activity. They will also help prevent injuries or injury recurrences. Following injury, they should be started as soon as they can be performed correctly, without pain. Pain should never be present during these exercises. The exercises can be done anywhere, and no special equipment is needed. These exercises should be performed 2 to 3 times a day, as long as the problem is present.

1. Pendulum Exercise

Standing with your feet apart, bend over at the waist. Fully extend your arms downward, and relax the shoulders. Move the shoulders and arms in small circles, gradually increasing the size of the circles. Then move the arms forward, back, left, and right **(Figure 15-9 and 10)**.

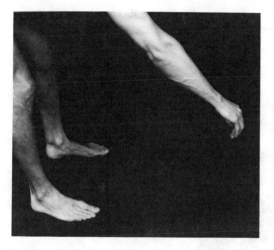

Figure 15-9.

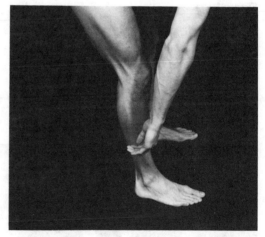

Figure 15-10.

2. Finger Wall Climb

Stand an arm's distance away from the wall. Walk the fingers of both hands up the wall until pain begins. Do this facing the wall **(Figure 15-11 and 12)**, then standing sideways to the wall for each arm **(Figure 15-13)**. Do this exercise 3 to 5 times, twice daily.

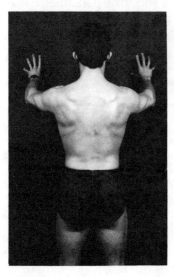 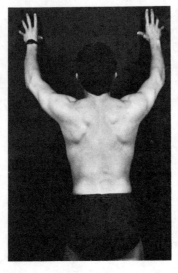 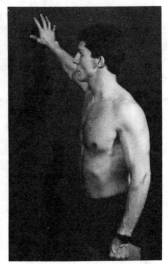

Figure 15-11.   **Figure 15-12.**   **Figure 15-13.**

3. Shoulder Stretching

a. Stand with one arm bent. With the opposite hand, grasp the elbow of your bent arm, and gently pull it across your body **(Figure 15-14 and 15)**. Hold 8 to 10 seconds, and relax. Repeat with the other arm. Do 5 to 8 times, twice daily.

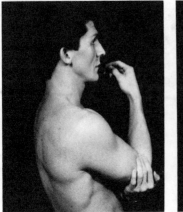 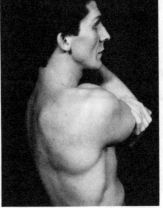

Figure 15-14.   **Figure 15-15.**

b. Stand with one arm bent over your head. With the opposite hand, grasp the bent elbow, and gently pull your arm down behind your head **(Figure 15-16)**. Hold 8 to 10 seconds and relax. Repeat with the other arm. Do 5 to 8 times, twice daily.

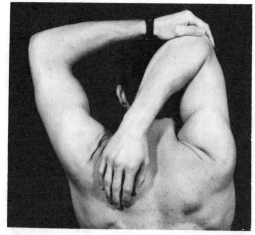

Figure 15-16.

4. Inward/Outward Shoulder Exercise

Sit with one arm bent at a 90-degree angle and your opposite hand across the chest, grasping your biceps **(Figure 15-17)**. Move bent arm inward, then move it outward as far as possible **(Figure 15-18 and 19)**. Do this in a slow, controlled manner. Do this 15 to 20 times, in each direction, twice daily. Repeat exercise with the other arm if you are working both shoulders. To make this exercise more difficult, hold a small weight.

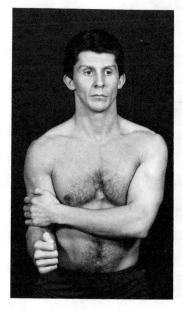

Figure 15-17.

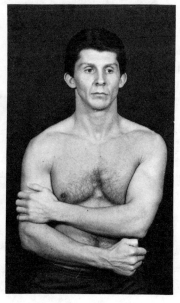

Figure 15-18.

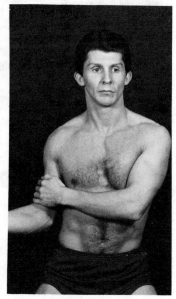

Figure 15-19.

5. Elevation Shoulder Exercise

a. Sit with your arms at your side (**Figure 15-20**). Raise one arm straight up, above your head (**Figure 15-21**). Lower it slowly. Do this exercise 15 to 20 times, twice daily. Repeat with the other arm if you are working both shoulders. To make this exercise more difficult, hold a small weight in the lifting hand.

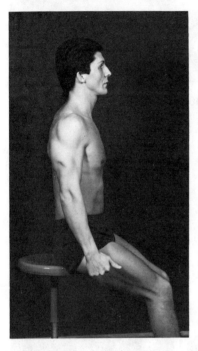

Figure 15-20.

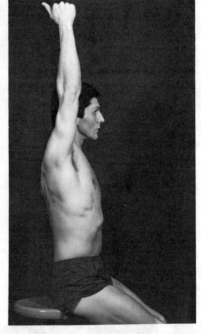

Figure 15-21.

b. Same as a, but raise the arm out to the side, stopping at shoulder level (**Figure 15-22 and 23**).

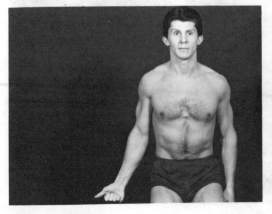

Figure 15-22.

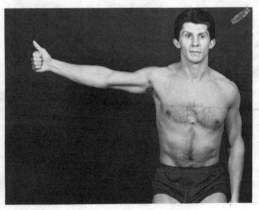

Figure 15-23.

6. Biceps Curl

Sit with one arm bent at a 90-degree angle **(Figure 15-24)**. Pull bent arm upward toward shoulder **(Figure 15-25)**. Do this 15 to 20 times, twice daily. Repeat with the other arm if you are working both shoulders. To make this exercise more difficult, hold a small weight in the lifted arm.

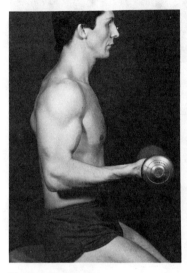
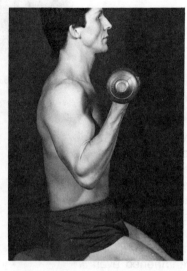

Figure 15-24.   **Figure 15-25.**

7. Triceps Exercise

Sit or stand with one elbow bent and pointing upward, with the hand dropped back **(Figure 15-26)**. Straighten the lower arm upward **(Figure 15-27)**. Repeat 15 to 20 times, twice daily. Do this exercise with the other arm if you are working both shoulders. To make this exercise more difficult, hold a small weight in the lifted arm.

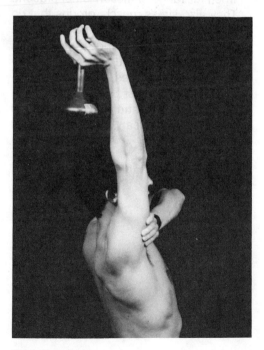

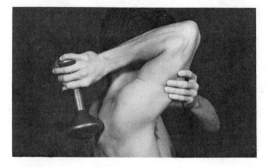

Figure 15-26.   **Figure 15-27.**

8. Push-ups

Lie on the floor, face down. Place your hands flat on floor, by your shoulders. Push the trunk straight upward, keeping your body in a straight line, extending the arms fully **(Figure 15-28)**. Return to the beginning position, touching only the chest to the floor, and repeat. Do 10 to 20 times, once a day.

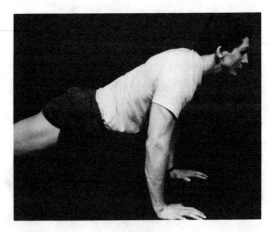

Figure 15-28.

9. Eccentric Loading Exercise

A type of exercise known as eccentric loading has proven to be extremely effective in the management of many chronic problems of the shoulder. This exercise series seems to relieve painful symptoms and hastens recovery time. Eccentric loading exercises emphasize a controlled range of motion, enabling the body part to be strengthened even when full range of motion is not present. They also stress muscle groups that do not perform the primary joint movement. The exercises restrengthen the area without risking re-injury or further overuse. These exercises (which are negative exercises) must be prescribed by a physician and taught by a physical therapist. They can be performed at home.

The Upper Arm

The muscles in the upper arm move the shoulder as well as the elbow. Therefore, many of the problems that occur in this area affect both the shoulder and the elbow. The most common injuries are muscle strains and bruises.

Chapter **16**

Discoloration
(Bruises, Contusions)

An upper arm contusion is usually the result of a direct blow to the outside of the arm **(Figure 16-1)**.

Symptoms

There is pain directly over the injured area. There may be some discoloration and local swelling. The muscles surrounding the injured area may be tight and/or stiff. Arm motion and especially elbow motion may be limited.

Do's

- Rest.
- Use ice, compression, and elevation.

Don'ts

- Do not massage the area.

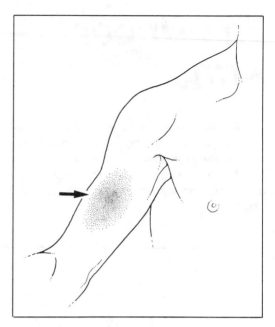

Figure 16-1. Upper arm contusion.

Modifications

- Pad the area if further contact is likely.
- Perform exercises 1 through 4 without pain.

Pulls (Strains)

Muscle pulls (strains) can occur in any muscle group in the body (see Chapter 1). Upper arm muscle strains **(Figure 16-2)** can be caused by overuse or sudden, vigorous activity.

Symptoms

There may be an area of specific pain directly over the affected muscle. You may feel pain in the muscle when you use the arm, or even when the arm is at rest. The area is usually stiff.

Do's

- Rest.
- Use ice, compression, and elevation.

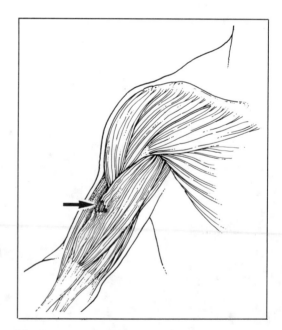

Figure 16-2. Muscle strain in upper arm.

Don'ts

- Do not perform activities that cause pain.

Modifications

- Do exercises 1 through 4 without pain.

Pain/Stiffness In Upper Arm
(Tendinitis in Upper Arm, Bicipital Tendinitis)

Bicipital tendinitis in the upper arm affects the biceps tendon, which attaches at the shoulder **(Figure 16-3)**. Usually it is caused by excessive pressure and/or repeated stress, as in excessive throwing or weight lifting.

Symptoms

The front of the shoulder aches, and there is pain when you move or work the muscle. A specific area of tenderness may be found directly over the inflammed tendon.

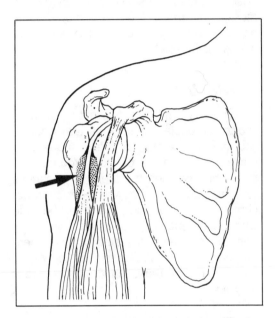

Figure 16-3. Biceps tendon—common location of tendinitis in the upper arm.

Do's

- Rest.
- Use ice and compression.

Don'ts

- Do not continue activities that are painful.

Modifications

- Do exercises 1 through 4 without pain. Exercise 2 may have to be deleted.

Total Tear Of Biceps Tendon
(Biceps Tendon Rupture)

In a biceps tendon rupture, the attachment pulls off and a portion of the muscle balls up, producing a "popeye muscle" **(Figure 16-4)**. If the rupture occurs at the opposite end of the muscle near the elbow, the muscle does not ball up. This problem can occur during very forceful, explosive movements, as in weight lifting.

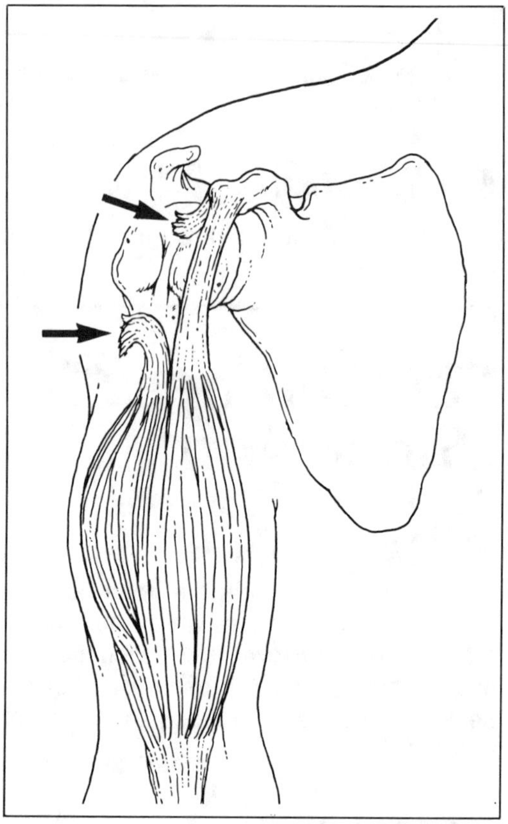

Symptoms

There is a muscle deformity known as "popeye muscle." When this tear occurs, you may hear a snap and feel sudden, intense pain at the site of injury. You can still move the shoulder, but there is weakness when you bend the elbow. If the rupture occurs at the elbow joint, there will be pain when you bend the elbow. You will know from the location of the area of pain where the tear occurred. A tear in the elbow usually requires surgery, but a shoulder tear may not.

Figure 16-4. Tear of biceps tendon.

Do's

- Rest.
- Use ice, compression, and elevation until there is less pain.
- See a physician.

Don'ts

- Do not continue any upper body activities until there is less pain.
- Do not do any activities that cause pain.

Modifications

- Do range of motion exercises for the shoulder and elbow.
- Do exercises 1 through 4 without pain if the rupture is from the shoulder.

Upper Arm Exercises

The following exercises should be used with the previous problems. They are designed to restrengthen the musculature that surrounds the injured area to hasten recovery and ensure a safe return to activity. They will also help prevent injuries or injury recurrences. Following injury, they should be started as soon as they can be performed correctly, without pain. Pain should never be present during these exercises. The exercises can be done anywhere, and no special equipment is needed. These exercises should be performed 2 to 3 times a day, as long as the problem is present.

1. Arm Stretching

a. Stand with your arm bent. With the opposite hand, grasp the elbow of your bent arm, and gently pull it across body **(Figure 16-5 and 6)**. Hold 8 to 10 seconds, and relax. Repeat with your other arm. Do 5 to 8 times, twice daily.

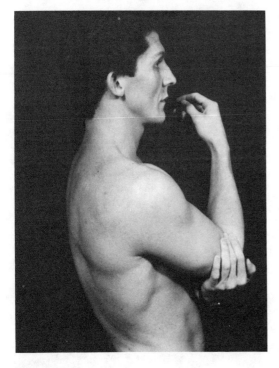

Figure 16-5.

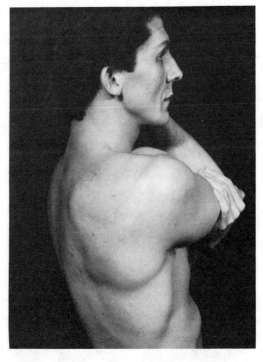

Figure 16-6.

b. Stand with one arm bent over your head. With the opposite hand, grasp the bent elbow, and gently pull your arm down behind your head **(Figure 16-7)**. Hold 8 to 10 seconds and relax. Repeat with the other arm. Do 5 to 8 times, twice daily.

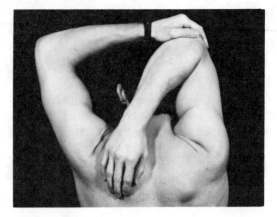

Figure 16-7.

2. *Biceps Curl*

Sit with one arm bent at a 90-degree angle **(Figure 16-8)**. Pull bent arm upward toward the shoulder **(Figure 16-9)**. Do this 15 to 20 times, twice daily. Repeat with the other arm. To make this exercise more difficult, hold small weight in the lifted arm.

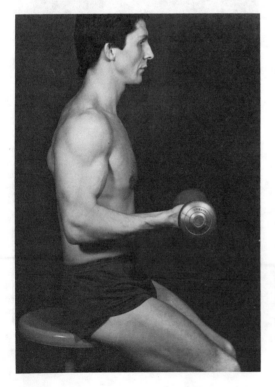

Figure 16-8.

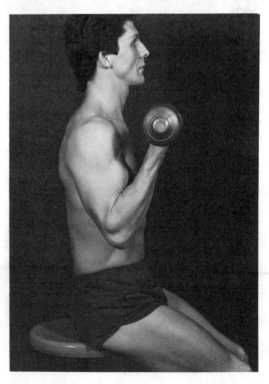

Figure 16-9.

3. Triceps Exercise

Sit or stand with one elbow bent and pointing upward, with the hand dropped back **(Figure 16-10)**. Straighten the bent arm upward **(Figure 16-11)**. Lower slowly. Do this 15 to 20 times, twice daily. Repeat with the other arm. To make this exercise more difficult, hold small weight in the lifted arm.

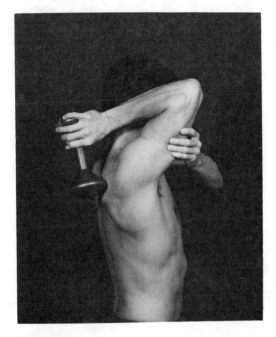

Figure 16-10.

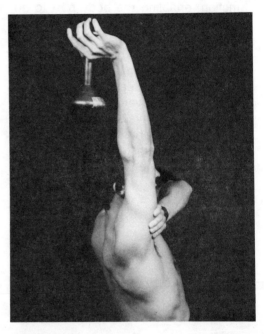

Figure 16-11.

4. Push-ups

Lie on the floor, face down. Place your hands flat on floor, by your shoulders. Push the trunk straight upward, keeping your body in a straight line, extending the arms fully **(Figure 16-12)**. Return to the beginning position, touching only the chest to the floor, and repeat. Do 10 to 20 times, once a day.

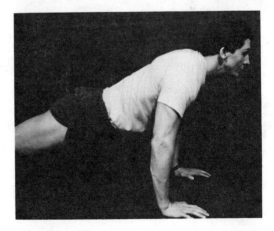

Figure 16-12.

5. Eccentric Loading Exercises

A type of rehabilitative exercise known as eccentric loading has proven to be extremely effective in the management of many chronic problems of the upper arm. This exercise series seems to relieve painful symptoms and hasten recovery time. Eccentric loading exercises emphasize a controlled limited range of motion, enabling the body part to be strengthened even when full range of motion is not present. They also stress muscle groups that do not perform the primary joint movement. The exercises restrengthen the area without risking reinjury or further overuse. The exercises (which are negative exercises) must be prescribed by a physician and taught by a physical therapist. They can be performed at home.

The Elbow

The muscles behind the elbow joint straighten it, and the muscles in front bend it. Injuries to the elbow can include ligament sprains and muscle strains.

Chapter *17*

Pain In Front Of Elbow
(Bicipital Tendinitis)

Bicipital tendinitis is an inflammation of the biceps muscle tendon where it attaches to the elbow **(Figure 17-1)**. This problem comes on gradually and may take several weeks to improve.

Symptoms

There is pain directly over the tendon area. There will be pain when you bend the elbow and/or when you pick up objects. It is also painful to turn the lower arm in and out. The area may ache at night.

Do's

- Rest.
- Use ice, compression, and elevation.

Don'ts

- Do not continue activities that are painful—the problem will get worse.

Modifications

- Use a sling if the problem is very painful.
- Do exercises 1 through 4 without pain.
- Eccentric loading exercises (see exercise 5) are *very* helpful.

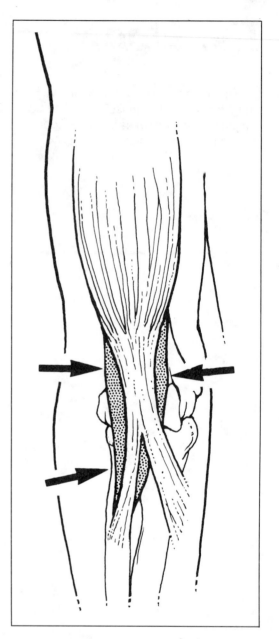

Figure 17-1. Inflammation of the biceps muscle tendon where it attaches to the elbow.

Pain When Elbow Straightens

(Elbow Hyperextension)

Hyperextension at the elbow joint (**Figure 17-2**) may occur at the elbow if the arm is forcefully pulled back or if you run into an immovable object with the arm straight. This injury may result in a ligament sprain as well as a muscle strain.

Symptoms

There is pain in the elbow joint especially as you try to fully straighten it. Full movement may not be possible. You will not be aware of just a single point of pain but rather a general aching throughout the joint. It may take several weeks for pain to disappear. You will feel more comfortable if you bend your elbow.

Do's

- Rest.
- Use ice, compression, and elevation.

Don'ts

- Do not perform any activities that cause pain.
- Do not force the arm to fully straighten.

Modifications

- Wear a sling if there is severe pain.
- Do exercises 1 through 4, without pain.
- As pain subsides over the next 3 to 6 weeks, check the elbow to see if it fully straightens. Do not let it get stuck in the bent position.

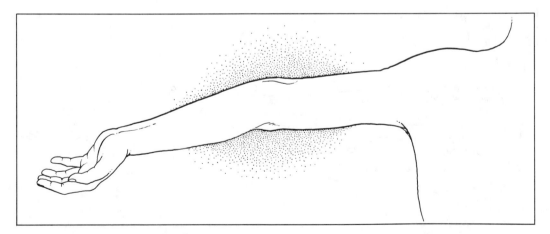

Figure 17-2. Hyperextension at the elbow joint.

Pain on Outside (Lateral) of Elbow

(Tennis Elbow, Lateral Epicondylitis)

The bony bump on the outside of the elbow **(Figure 17-3)** serves as an attachment for muscles which go down the forearm into the wrist. Through repeated stress, some fibers of these muscles may become irritated and pull off their attachments. While the condition is commonly called "tennis elbow" because it has resulted from playing tennis, it can occur with any sport or exercise. Tennis elbow occurs gradually and may take several months or year to heal.

Symptoms

There is a specific area of tenderness directly over the bony bump on the outside of the elbow. An aching sensation will be noticeable in the elbow and down into the forearm. You will experience pain when the arm and elbow are straight and the palm rotates upward and downward. It is especially painful to pick up objects. There may be limited motion of the elbow joint, only because of pain.

Do's

- Rest.
- Use ice, compression, and elevation.

Don'ts

- Do not continue activities that are painful, for the condition will get worse.

Modifications

- Wear a sling if pain is intense.
- Use a tennis elbow support at all times, even when you sleep, if it helps **(Figure 17-4)**.
- Do exercises 1 through 4, without pain.
- Eccentric loading (see exercise 5) is the treatment of choice.

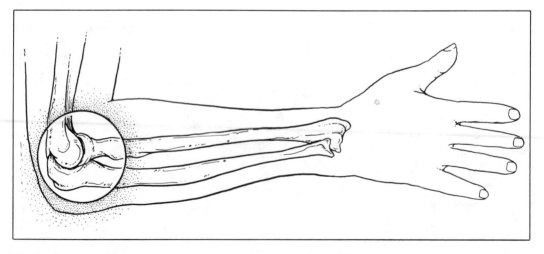

Figure 17-3. Bony bump in outside of elbow where "tennis elbow" usually occurs.

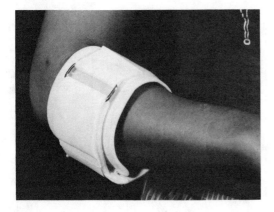

Figure 17-4. Tennis elbow support.

Pain on Inside of Elbow
(Medial Epicondylitis)

Pain on the inside of the elbow involves the muscles that attach on the inner elbow and go down the forearm to the wrist. Because of repeated stress, these muscles can be irritated where they attach to the elbow. This problem comes on gradually and may take several months to heal.

Symptoms

There is an area of pain directly over the muscle attachment **(Figure 17-5)**. Some minor swelling may be present. Motion at the elbow may be limited. You will experience pain when you twist the forearm by turning the palm of the hand, especially when you pick up objects.

Do's

- Rest.
- Use ice, compression, and elevation.

Don'ts

- Do not do any acitivities that are painful—this problem will get worse.

Modifications

- Use a sling if pain is severe.
- Do exercises 1 through 4, without pain.

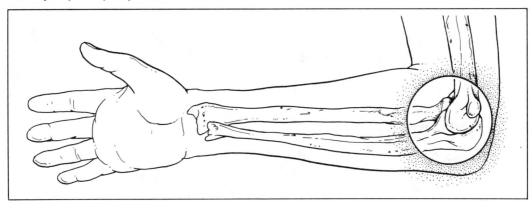

Figure 17-5. Location of pain on inside of the elbow, where muscles attach to bony bump.

Sudden Pain and Locking of Elbow
(Osteochondritis Dissecans, Pitcher's Elbow)

Repeated stress and/or trauma to the elbow, as in excessive throwing, may cause a small piece of bone or cartilage to break off in the joint **(Figure 17-6)**. This can occur on the outside or inside of the elbow, deep within the joint. There will be symptoms in the elbow long before the piece comes loose, so preventive actions are advisable.

Symptoms

Activities such as throwing cause pain that can be relieved with rest. Excessive use increases the pain, and if the problem continues, pain persists even with rest. The elbow may become locked if the bone fragment becomes loose and lodged between the bones. Sudden pain will be experienced when this occurs. There may be some swelling in the area, which you can feel more than you can see.

Do's

- Rest.
- Use ice, compression, and elevation.

Don'ts

- Do not continue throwing motions. This will only make the bony fragments come loose.
- Avoid activities that cause pain.

Modifications

- Continue lower extremity exercises.
- If locking continues, you will need to see a physician.

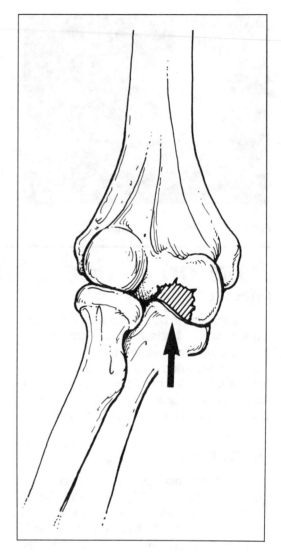

Figure 17-6. Small piece of bone or cartilage broken off in elbow.

Swelling Behind Elbow
(Elbow Bursitis, Olecranon Bursitis)

An injured bursa in the elbow is often located directly at the back of the joint, almost at the point of the elbow **(Figure 17-7)**. Usually it becomes injured from a direct blow to the elbow in contact sports, as in falling on the turf in football.

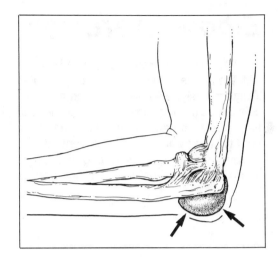

Figure 17-7. Injured and inflamed bursa at point of elbow.

Symptoms

There is pain and visible, immediate swelling directly in the area of the bursa. It may be hard to bend the elbow.

Do's

- Rest.
- Use ice, compression, and elevation.

Don'ts

- Do not continue throwing or lifting movements.

Modifications

- Pad the elbow if it is likely to be hit again.

Elbow Exercises

The following exercises should be used with the problems discussed in this chapter. They are designed to restrengthen the musculature that surrounds the injured area to hasten recovery and ensure a safe return to activity. They will also help prevent injuries or injury recurrences. Following injury, they should be started as soon as they can be performed correctly, without pain. Pain should never be present during these exercises. The exercises can be done anywhere, and no special equipment is needed. These exercises should be performed 2 to 3 times a day, as long as the problem is present.

---

1. Biceps Curl

Sit with one arm bent at a 90-degree angle **(Figure 17-8)**. Pull the bent arm upward toward the shoulder **(Figure 17-9)**. Do this 15 to 20 times, twice daily. Repeat with the other arm. To make this exercise more difficult, hold a small weight in the lifted arm.

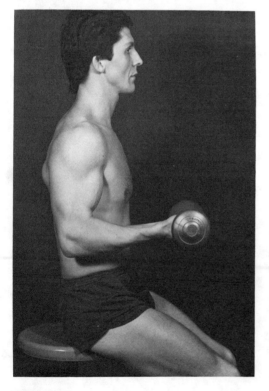

Figure 17-8.

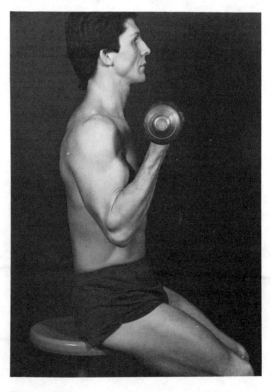

Figure 17-9.

2. Triceps Exercise

Sit or stand with one elbow bent and pointing upward, with the hand dropped back **(Figure 17-10)**. Straighten the bent arm upward **(Figure 17-11)**. Lower slowly. Repeat 15 to 20 times, twice daily. Do this exercise with the other arm if you are working both elbows. To make this exercise more difficult, hold a small weight in the lifted arm.

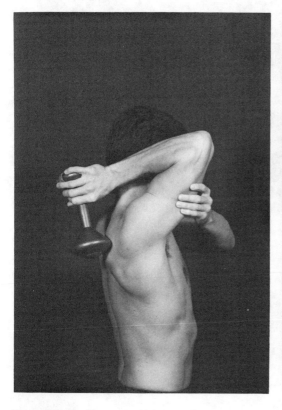

Figure 17-10.

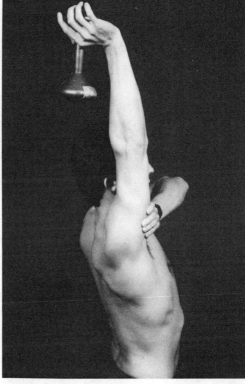

Figure 17-11.

3. Push-ups

Lie on the floor, face down. Place your hands flat on floor, by your shoulders. Push the trunk straight upward, keeping your body in a straight line, extending the arms fully **(Figure 17-12)**. Return to the beginning position, touching only the chest to the floor, and repeat. Do 10 to 20 times, once a day.

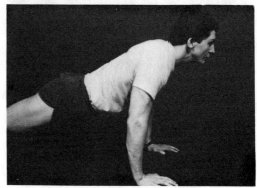

Figure 17-12.

4. Towel Twist

Stand or sit, and hold a towel between your hands. Twist the towel with both hands, forward and backward **(Figure 17-13)**. Do this exercise 10 to 15 times, twice daily.

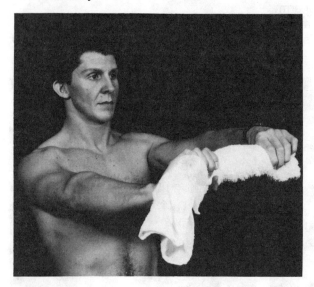

Figure 17-13.

5. Eccentric Loading Exercise

A type of exercise known as eccentric loading has proven to be extremely effective in the management of many chronic problems of the elbow. This exercise seems to relieve painful symptoms and hasten recovery time. Eccentric loading exercises emphasize a controlled range of motion, enabling the body part to be strengthened even when full range of motion is not present. They also stress muscle groups that do not perform the primary joint movement. The exercises restrengthen the area without risking re-injury or further overuse. These exercises (which are negative exercises) must be prescribed by a physician and taught by a physical therapist. They can be performed at home.

The Wrist and Fingers

The wrist contains many bones and ligaments through which nerves, vessels, and tendons pass from the forearm to the hand and fingers **(Figure 18-1)**. Each finger contains bones, ligaments across the joints, tendons to straighten and bend the fingers, arteries, veins, and nerves. Multiple problems can occur and should be considered serious.

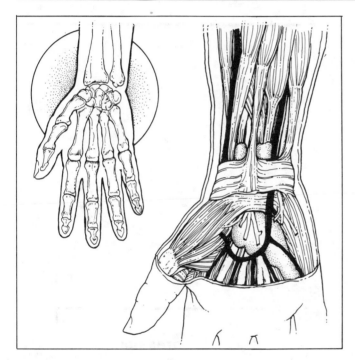

Figure 18-1. Bones, ligaments, nerves, vessels, and tendons of the wrist and hand.

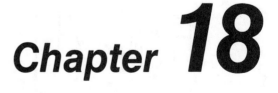

Chapter **18**

Pain Traveling Down Wrist/Hand
(Nerve Compression in Wrist —Carpal Tunnel Syndrome, Ulnar Tunnel Syndrome)

Nerves traveling through the wrist to the palm of the hand and fingers must pass through very narrow spaces or tunnels. Sometimes a nerve becomes trapped or compressed in one of these tunnels, which causes pain in the wrist and tingling in the fingers **(Figure 18-2)**.

Symptoms

Carpal Tunnel Syndrome is characterized by aching pain in the wrist, and sharp, burning pain, tingling, and weakness in the thumb, index finger, middle finger, and half of the ring finger. You may shake your hand to relieve the problem.

Ulnar Tunnel Syndrome will cause tingling in the 2 little fingers. It is very important to know which fingers are involved. (See Ulnar Neuropathy later in this chapter.)

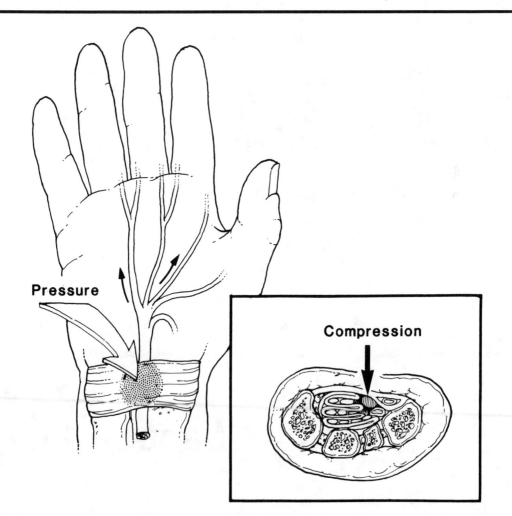

Pressure

Compression

Figure 18-2. Compressed nerve in wrist, causing pain in wrist and tingling in fingers (Carpal Tunnel Syndrome).

Do's

- Rest.
- Use ice, compression, and elevation.
- Wear wrist splint with the wrist out straight **(Figure 18-3)**.

Don'ts

- Do not keep wrist in bent down position for long periods of time.
- Do not continue activities that cause pain.

Modifications

- A splint to hold the wrist in a straight or slightly bent-up position may help.

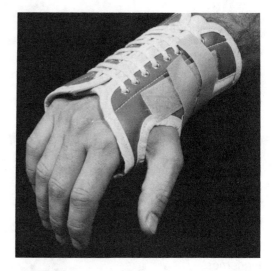

Figure 18-3. Wrist splint.

Weakness and Tingling in Ring and Little Fingers
(Handlebar Palsy, Ulnar Neuropathy)

This problem is caused by pressure on the ulnar nerve, which goes to the ring finger and little finger. The condition can occur in one or both hands. Usually pressure is caused by gripping the handlebars of a bike tightly or leaning on the hands in the same position for a long time.

Symptoms

There is pain, tingling, and numbness in the ring and little fingers. Other possible symptoms are weakness throughout the hand and a loss of coordination.

Do's

- Change your hand position frequently when biking.
- Wear padded gloves.
- Check handlebar height on your bike.

Don'ts

- Don't ignore this problem, as it may cause permanent nerve damage.

Modifications

- Do all exercises with caution unless weakness persists, in which case you should see a physician.

Sprained Wrist

A sprain to the ligaments in the wrist usually occurs when you fall on an out-stretched hand or cause forced movement in the wrist. Be careful—a minor sprain to the wrist is usually a major problem.

Symptoms

There is general pain in the wrist area, usually over the top of the joint. Swelling is present throughout the joint. Movement is limited, and the wrist may feel weak at times. There is no specific point of pain and tenderness.

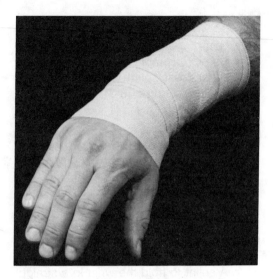

Figure 18-4. Compression bandage.

Do's

- Rest.
- Use ice, compression, and elevation.
- See a physician.

Don'ts

- Do not continue activities that cause pain.
- Do not forcefully grip or grasp anything.

Modifications

If cleared by a physician:
- Wear a compression bandage to provide support **(Figure 18-4)**.
- Do exercises 1 through 4, without pain.

Sharp Pain In Wrist
(Broken Bone in Wrist— Navicular Fracture)

The most commonly fractured bone in the wrist is the navicular bone, located on the thumb side **(Figure 18-5)**. The fracture usually occurs when you fall on an out-stretched hand. This problem is often mistaken for a sprained wrist. You must carefully observe the symptoms to identify the injury.

Symptoms

There is pain in the wrist. You will notice muscle weakness. Usually there is a specific area of tenderness directly over the navicular bone **(Figure 18-6)**. You will notice pain if you apply upward pressure to the long bone in the thumb.

Do's

- Rest.
- Use ice, compression, and elevation.
- See a physician. If the navicular bone is broken, you will need surgery or a cast.

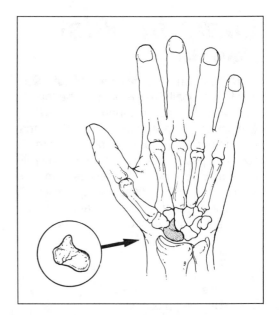

Figure 18-5. Location of most commonly fractured bone in the wrist— the navicular bone.

Don'ts

- Do not continue activities that cause pain.
- Do not bend or straighten the wrist.

Modifications

- See a physician for an accurate diagnosis.
- Continue all other conditioning.

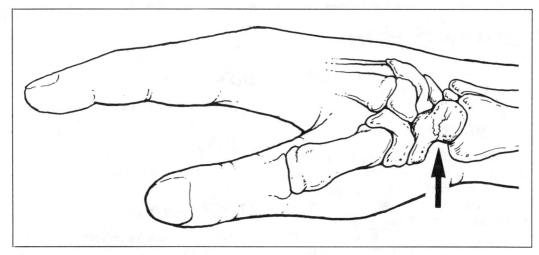

Figure 18-6. Area of tenderness over navicular bone if bone is fractured.

Lump in Wrist
(Wrist Ganglion)

A ganglion is a small mass of soft tissue that forms a ball-like swelling on the top of a joint, very close to the surface **(Figure 18-7)**. A wrist ganglion appears slowly and may follow an injury. The mass ranges from the size of a pea to the size of a large marble, and it may get bigger. Pain results from pressure on surrounding tissue or constant irritation. If the ganglion is surgically removed, there is a good chance of recurrence.

Do's

- Use ice.
- Use compression.

Don'ts

- Try not to irritate or hit the area.

Modifications

- Apply mild pressure to the area with a small foam pad taped over the ganglion **(Figure 18-8)**.
- See a physician to confirm that the lump is indeed a ganglion or if the ganglion becomes larger.

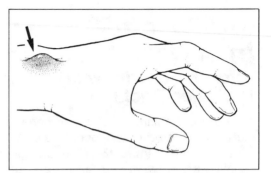

Figure 18-7. Small mass of soft tissue in wrist—wrist ganglion.

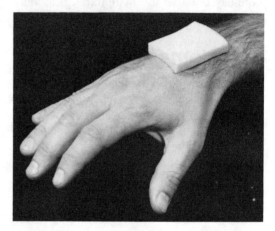

Figure 18-8. Ganglion pad.

Bruised Hand

Bruises usually occur on the back or the palm side of the hand.

Symptoms

There is discoloration and tenderness directly over the area where contact was made. Some swelling may be present in the bruised area. You may notice pain when you move the wrist and fingers.

Do's

- Use ice, compression, and elevation.

Don'ts

- Do not do activities that cause pain.

Modifications

- Pad the area for protection if contact is likely.

Fractures

Fractures may occur in any bone of the wrist, hand, or fingers **(Figure 18-9)**. Usually a specific incident caused the fracture.

Symptoms

There is pain directly over the fracture site. Swelling is present around the area. It will be very painful and difficult to move the injured area, which may look deformed.

Do's

- See a physician.
- Rest.
- Use ice, compression, and elevation.

Don'ts

- Do not move the injured area.

Modifications

- Continue all other activities.
- After the fracture has healed, do exercises 1 through 4, without pain.

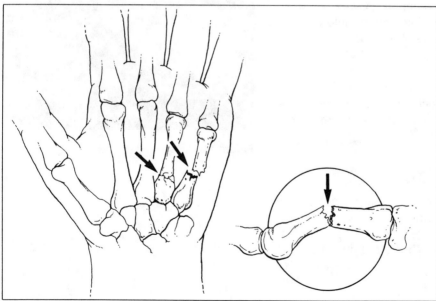

Figure 18-9. Fractures in the bones of the hand.

Pain in Fingers
(Finger Sprains, Dislocated Finger Joints)

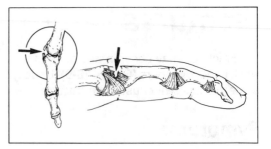

Sprains often occur in the ligaments of the fingers **(Figure 18-10)**. They are caused by forceful movements or contact that pushes the finger in a direction in which it is not supposed to go. Frequent sprains may cause permanent enlargement of the knuckles. It is essential to treat finger sprains promptly and properly. Remember it takes 6 weeks to heal a ligament. If you do not protect the injury adequately, the problem will remain for life.

Figure 18-10. Sprains in a ligament of a finger.

Symptoms

There is general pain and swelling in the injured area. The finger will be stiff and difficult to bend and straighten. Some discoloration may be present. A joint may be separated or dislocated.

Do's

- If a joint is dislocated, see a physician.
- Use ice, compression, and elevation.
- Splint the injured finger onto the next finger if possible **(Figure 18-11)**.

Don'ts

- Do not continue to move the finger unless it is supported by the other fingers.

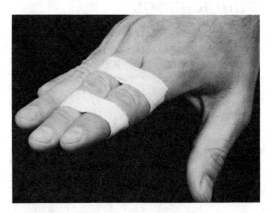

Figure 18-11. Splinted fingers.

Modifications

- Perform activities that do not involve the injured area.
- Use adhesive tape to support the finger with another finger during activity.
- Do exercises 1 through 4, without pain.

Thumb Sprain
(Gamekeeper's Thumb, Skier's Thumb)

A sprain to the ligaments of the thumb is caused by falling on the hand with the thumb outstretched away from the hand **(Figure 18-12)**. This tears the ligament on the inside of the thumb and produces looseness in that joint.

Symptoms

There is specific pain and tenderness on the side of the big knuckle of the thumb, closest to the hand. Swelling may be present. You will notice pain when you move the thumb and try to grasp something. There will also be weakness when you grasp.

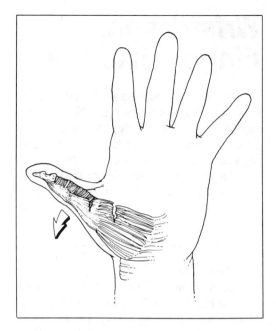

Figure 18-12. Thumb sprain.

Do's

- Rest.
- Use ice, compression, and elevation.
- This can be a serious, life-long problem. It should be evaluated by a physician.

Don'ts

- Do not continue to try to use your thumb—it will only make the problem worse.

Modifications

- Tape the injured area. **(Figure 18-13)**.
- Do exercises 1 through 4, without pain.

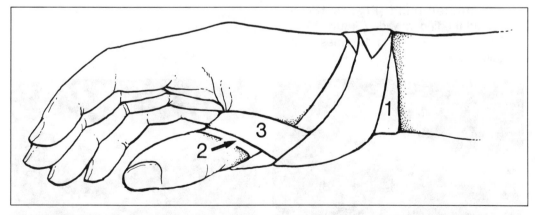

Figure 18-13. *Thumb taping:* Using 1-inch adhesive tape (1) circle the wrist and begin a figure-8 pattern around the large joint of the thumb, (2) and (3). Repeat the pattern at least 3 times or until joint is covered.

Wrist/Hand/ Finger Exercises

The following exercises should be used with the previous problems. They are designed to restrengthen the musculature that surrounds the injured area to hasten recovery and ensure a safe return to activity. They will also help prevent injuries or injury recurrences. Following injury, they should be started as soon as they can be performed correctly, without pain. Pain should never be present during these exercises. The exercises can be done anywhere, and no special equipment is needed. These exercises should be performed 2 to 3 times a day, as long as the problem is present.

---

1. Towel Twist

Stand or sit, and hold a towel between your hands. Twist the towel forward and backward **(Figure 18-14)**. Do this exercise 10 to 15 times, twice daily.

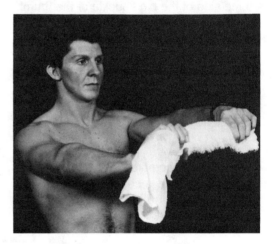

Figure 18-14.

2. Grip and Spread

Stand or sit, and make a tight fist with your injured hand **(Figure 18-15)**. Spread the fingers wide **(Figure 18-16)**. Do this exercise 10 to 15 times, twice daily.

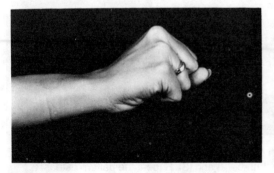

Figure 18-15.

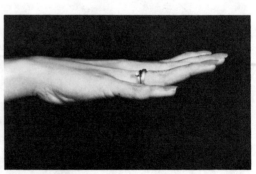

Figure 18-16.

3. Grip and Squeeze

Stand or sit, and hold a squeezable elastic bandage in your injured hand **(Figure 18-17)**. Squeeze it tightly, and relax **(Figure 18-18)**. Do this exercise 10 to 15 times, twice daily.

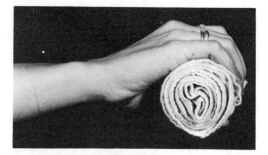

Figure 18-17.

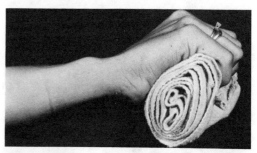

Figure 18-18.

4. Wrist Curl Flexion/Extension

a. Sit with your arm on a table or desk, bent at a 90-degree angle, with your hand over the edge, palm up. Hold a small 1- to 5-pound weight in your injured hand **(Figure 18-19)**. Bend the hand toward your arm (flexion) **(Figure 18-20)**, then straighten the hand out and away from your arm (extension) **(Figure 18-21)**. Do this exercise 10 to 15 times, twice daily.

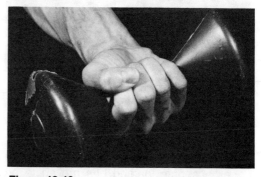

Figure 18-19.

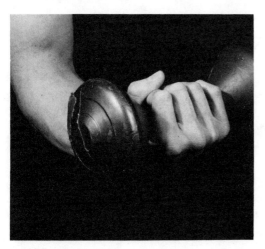

Figure 18-20.

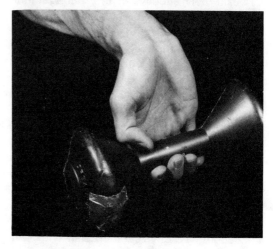

Figure 18-21.

b. Same as above with palm down **(Figure 18-22, 23 and 24)**.

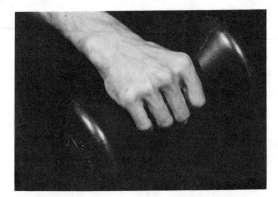

Figure 18-22.

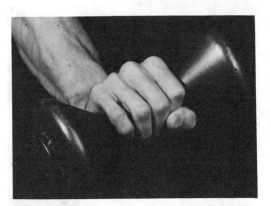

Figure 18-23.

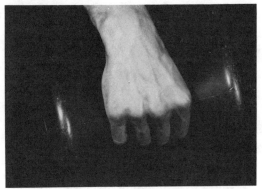

Figure 18-24.

5. *Eccentric Loading Exercises*

A type of rehabilitative exercise known as eccentric loading has proven to be extremely effective in the management of many chronic problems of the wrist. This exercise series seems to relieve painful symptoms and hasten recovery time. Eccentric loading exercises emphasize a controlled limited range of motion, enabling the body part to be strengthened even when full range of motion is not present. They also stress muscle groups that do not perform the primary joint movement. The exercises restrengthen the area without risking reinjury or further overuse. These exercises (which are negative exercises) must be prescribed by a physician and taught by a physical therapist. They can be performed at home.

About the Authors

Merrill A. Ritter, M.D., is professor of orthopedics at Indiana University Medical Center. He is also medical director of the Center for Hip and Knee Surgery in Mooresville, Indiana. He holds degrees from Kenyon College in Gambier, Ohio, and the Indiana University School of Medicine. A prominent orthopedic surgeon, specializing in sports medicine and total joint replacement, Dr. Ritter has published more than 100 articles in professional journals and presented numerous papers at medical meetings throughout the world. He is a leader in the research and development of artificial joint replacement devices and innovative knee ligament reconstruction procedures. Dr. Ritter has served as orthopedic surgeon for the athletic teams at Indiana University in Bloomington, Indiana, for 13 years. He served on the medical committee for the 1987 Pan American Games. He has chaired the Sports Medicine Committee of the United States Gymnastics Federation and was chief medical officer for the 1987 World Indoor Track and Field Championship.

Marjorie Albohm, A.T., C., is a faculty member at the Indiana University School of Medicine. She received her bachelor's degree from Valparaiso University in Valparaiso, Indiana, and master's degree from Indiana State University in physical education, with a speciality in athletic training. She was one of the first women in the nation to be certified by the National Athletic Trainers Association. Ms. Albohm has published articles appearing in numerous professional journals and has previously written a book titled *Health Care and the Female Athlete.* She has also been on the medical staff for several international events, including the 1979 World University Games in Mexico City and the 1980 Winter Olympic Games in Lake Placid. An accomplished speaker and lecturer, Ms. Albohm has presented numerous programs on various topics in sports medicine throughout the nation. She has received many awards of recognition, the most recent being the Distinguished Service Award of the National Interscholastic Athletic Administrators Association. Ms. Albohm was a member of the medical services committee and a community fitness committee for the 1987 Pan American Games and chaired the medical committee for the 1987 World Indoor Track and Field Championships.